WALKING SALT LAKE CITY

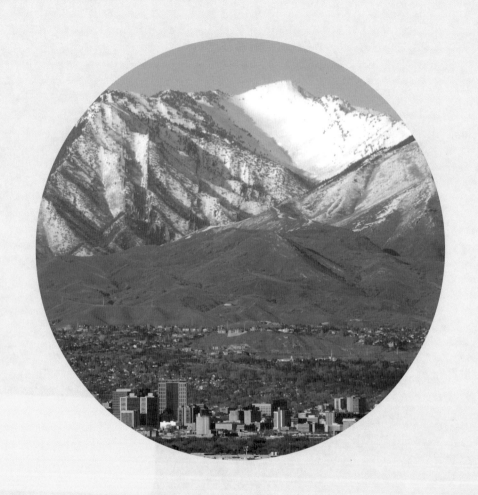

WALKING
SALT LAKE CITY

At the Crossroads of the West,
34 Tours Spotlight Urban Paths, Historic
Architecture, Forgotten Places, and
Religious and Cultural Icons

Lynn Arave & Ray Boren

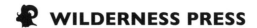 **WILDERNESS PRESS**

Walking Salt Lake City: At the Crossroads of the West, 34 Tours Spotlight Urban Paths, Historic Architecture, Forgotten Places, and Religious and Cultural Icons

1st EDITION 2012

Copyright © 2012 by Lynn Arave and Ray Boren

Cover and interior photos copyright © Ray Boren
Maps: Scott McGrew
Cover and book design: Larry B. Van Dyke and Lisa Pletka
Book layout: Annie Long
Book editor: Holly Cross
ISBN 978-0-89997-692-1

Manufactured in the United States of America

Published by: **Wilderness Press**
Keen Communications
PO Box 43673
Birmingham, AL 35243
(800) 443-7227; FAX (205) 326-1012
info@wildernesspress.com
www.wildernesspress.com

Visit our website for a complete listing of our books and for ordering information.

Distributed by Publishers Group West

Cover photos: *Front, clockwise from top left:* Temple Square, as seen from the top of the Conference Center (Walk 1); Utah State Capitol (Walk 6); Salt Lake City skyline, from the southwest; Salt Lake Temple, Temple Square (Walk 1); Main Library/Library Square (Walk 4); Utah State Capitol at sunset, from the east (Walk 6, as viewed from Walk 14, Upper Avenues); This Is the Place Monument at This Is the Place Heritage Park (Walk 20); *Back, clockwise from top right:* Memory Grove/City Creek in autumn (Walk 7); Madonna wall mural, downtown Salt Lake City (Walk 4); Richards Street fountains, City Creek Center, City Center (Walk 3).

SAFETY NOTICE: Although Wilderness Press and the authors have made every attempt to ensure that the information in this book is accurate at press time, they are not responsible for any loss, damage, injury, or inconvenience that may occur to anyone while using this book. You are responsible for your own safety and health while following the walking trips described here. Always check local conditions, know your own limitations, and consult a map.

To our parents, Gene S. and Norma R. Arave and Don L. and Phyllis Ottley Boren, who bequeathed to us a wonderful sense of place.

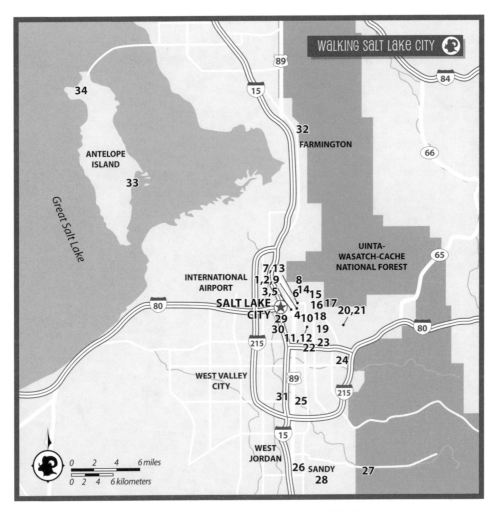

NUMBERS ON THIS LOCATOR MAP CORRESPOND TO WALK NUMBERS.

acknowledgments

No less a figure than Albert Einstein is credited with saying "The distinction between the past, present, and future is only a stubbornly persistent illusion." The great theorist may have been contemplating the nature of "time" itself, but his words seem evocative when strolling through the history-laced neighborhoods and business districts of today's Salt Lake City and Salt Lake Valley. Past, present, and future mingle on such walks. Because of this effect, the authors gratefully acknowledge the research and tales that unfold for the general public in books and pamphlets, on the Web, and on historic markers and plaques by such organizations as the Utah Heritage Foundation, the Utah State Historical Society and Utah Division of State History, the Daughters of Utah Pioneers, and Sons of Utah Pioneers. As for the present, in a city undergoing remarkable change, the authors thank the City Creek Center, Intrepid Group, and specifically Dee Brewer, Leigh Dethman, Ronald A. Loch, and Linda S. Wardell, for tours and updates that have helped make the information presented here as fresh as can be. We also thank our editors, Susan Haynes and Holly Cross, and their staff, for their guidance, scrutiny, and patience. Finally, we credit author Greg Witt, who recommended us to Wilderness Press as authors for this book.

author's note

Nestled in a high valley where the rumpled Great Basin of the American West meets the first ramparts of the Rocky Mountains, people in Salt Lake City experience all four seasons. And perhaps a few more, for the edges of winter and spring can certainly be a bit fuzzy, giving us "sprinter," for example. The shift from autumn into winter takes its time, as well, offering changes day to day—until the real snow, fog, and, yes, smog, settle into place. Particularly annoying are stretches when a high pressure aloft puts a cap atop the Salt Lake Valley, allowing particulates to accumulate in the trapped, cold air, while slightly warmer conditions and bluer skies prevail in higher valleys and at the tops of canyons, where Utah's famous ski resorts offer an escape. That said, walking is possible in all of Salt Lake City's seasons; just beware of seasonal ice and snow and avoid lowland treks on unhealthy "red burn" days in winter.

Some visitors are also initially confused by the Salt Lake Valley's street grid and numbering system. Certain streets have formal names (State Street, Main Street, Martin Luther King

Boulevard), but all also have a number. The designations are usually in the hundreds (100 South is also known as First South), with building addresses filling in the difference. The grid system's ground zero is at Main and South Temple Streets, the southeast corner of the Mormon pioneers' original Temple Square. From there, going west, for instance, one comes to West Temple (100 West) and onward to 200 West, 300 West, and so on. State Street is 100 East, with 200 East, 300 East, and so on, continuing eastward. South Temple and Main Streets are "zeroes." So, for instance, 100 South is one block to South Temple's south, and the numbering system continues unfurling toward, for instance, 120th South (12000 South) in Draper and Riverton on the valley's other end.

State and street maps, as well as guides to local attractions, are available at information centers, such as the Utah Travel Council offices across from the Utah State Capitol and the Salt Lake Convention and Visitors Bureau in the Calvin L. Rampton Salt Palace Convention Center. They are well worth a visit for orientation and advice.

TABLE OF CONTENTS

INTRODUCTION

Salt Lake City is a Western American metropolis like no other. Events, personalities, and architecture of a century (and more!) seem to hover over the here and now. The city was founded in 1847 by religious refugees, the Mormons—more properly, members of The Church of Jesus Christ of Latter-day Saints. The community predates the Gold Rush and California's quick statehood. There was no Denver, and no Colorado, for that matter. Western Missouri was the frontier; the mislabeled "Great American Desert," the Rocky Mountains, and hundreds of miles intervened between the United States proper and the Pacific Coast. However, the Mormons' new Zion did not long remain the isolated kingdom they sought. The lure of gold soon propelled thousands upon thousands of Forty-Niners toward California. Then came stagecoaches, the Pony Express, the Transcontinental Railroad, and modern highways, as well as non-Mormon merchants and miners. Salt Lake City became "the Crossroads of the West."

Walking Salt Lake City is a time-traveling guide to both that past and the vibrant present. Written by Utah natives, it presents rambles of every kind. The 34 tours explore the city's downtown, which is experiencing an invigorating renaissance; Temple Square, world headquarters of the LDS Church; Capitol Hill; character-filled neighborhoods like the Avenues and "15th and 15th"; and semi-rural surprises near and within the bustling city, from Memory Grove and City Creek Canyon, a stone's throw from metropolitan skyscrapers, to tucked-away and nearly forgotten Miller Bird Preserve and the appropriately named Hidden Hollow.

While snow-capped mountains, famous canyon resorts, and the inland sea that gave the city its name invitingly beckon hikers, skiers, snowboarders, climbers, and day-trippers, *Walking Salt Lake City* unveils tempting reasons to enjoy the urban setting itself. Thoughtfully designed, the guide offers precise directions, easy-to-follow summaries, and tips about inviting eateries and shopping havens. Whether you are out for a heart-pumping workout or an evening stroll, filling an hour or a day, or count yourself a Utah visitor, a new resident, or a lifelong local, this book is designed with you in mind. *Walking Salt Lake City* is part of a national book series that details walking routes in key U.S. cities. The guide is geared so a reader can pick it up, choose an area to stroll, and quickly be out on the sidewalk doing

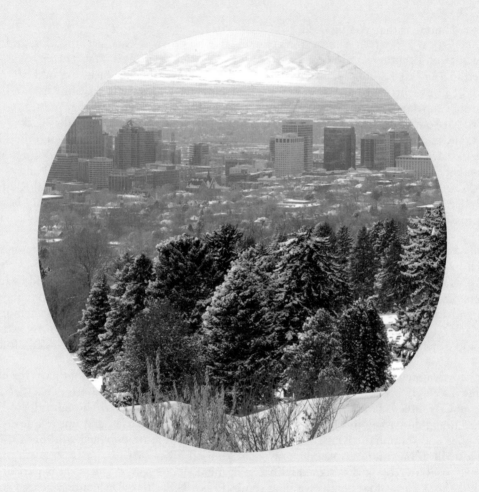

Downtown Salt Lake City

exactly that. Descriptions and turn-by-turn directions make it a breeze to use. That said, the city and its surroundings offer even more options. The chapters that follow may entice you to explore adjacent streets and neighborhoods, and who could blame you?

Our sincere hope is that you will relish the history, tales, and details about places you wish to discover, or may have thought you knew, and will be surprised about ideas for walks you may not have considered before.

Also, realize that this book contains just a sampling of possible walks that could be taken in the greater Salt Lake City area.

Enjoy!

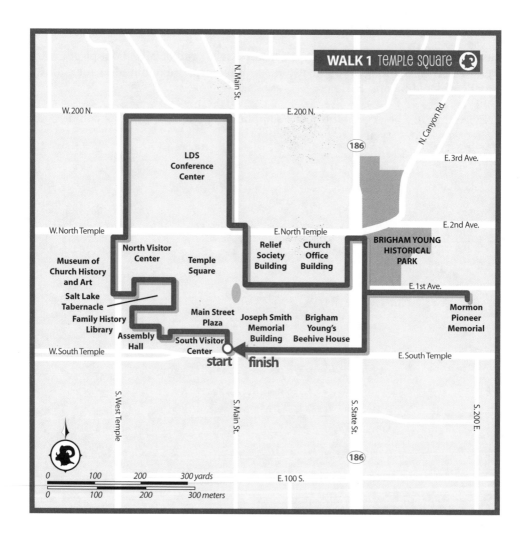

WALK 1 TEMPLE SQUARE

W. 200 N.

E. 200 N.

N. Main St.

N. Canyon Rd.

186

E. 3rd Ave.

LDS Conference Center

E. 2nd Ave.

W. North Temple

E. North Temple

BRIGHAM YOUNG HISTORICAL PARK

North Visitor Center

Relief Society Building

Church Office Building

Museum of Church History and Art

Temple Square

E. 1st Ave.

Salt Lake Tabernacle

Mormon Pioneer Memorial

Family History Library

Main Street Plaza

Joseph Smith Memorial Building

Brigham Young's Beehive House

Assembly Hall

South Visitor Center

W. South Temple

E. South Temple

start **finish**

S. West Temple

S. Main St.

S. State St.

S. 200 E.

186

0   100   200   300 yards

0   100   200   300 meters

E. 100 S.

1 Temple Square: The Mormon "Mecca"

BOUNDARIES: South Temple, West Temple, 200 North, and 200 East
DISTANCE: 2 miles (serpentine and approximate)
DIFFICULTY: Easy
PARKING: Beneath the Joseph Smith Memorial Building via South Temple and beneath City Creek Center (fees) or curbside (metered)
PUBLIC TRANSIT: TRAX light-rail's City Center and Temple Square stops–the former a half block south of Temple Square on Main St., the latter one block west on South Temple–are near our starting point. Bus and TRAX rides cost nothing within the downtown Free Fare Zone.

Prayers and pilgrimages point Muslims to Mecca; Hindus and Buddhists to Varanasi on the sacred River Ganges; Catholics to Rome; and Jews, Christians, and Muslims all toward Jerusalem. While members of The Church of Jesus Christ of Latter-day Saints (LDS)—the Mormons—share the holy places of Christendom, Salt Lake City is their "Mecca," and at the very heart of the religion is Temple Square. In his travelogue/reminiscence of the 1860s, *Roughing It,* Mark Twain nicknamed this city "the stronghold of the prophets." Once describing a single, walled 10-acre city block, today the Temple Square campus embraces not only the iconic LDS Temple and oval Salt Lake Tabernacle but also the church's world headquarters, located in multiple structures, including a skyscraper. A huge conference center has risen across the way. The church's renowned genealogy library and museum beckon to the west. And in the midst of all this are the 160-year-old homes and offices of Brigham Young, known to some as the American Moses. In 1847 he led his harassed people into the wilderness that was the Mountain West. A meander through all of this can occupy less than an hour. Or, by taking advantage of free tours on Temple Square proper or in the many LDS buildings, you can make it a half-day or even a full-day excursion—or more.

● Let's begin at Salt Lake City's topographical keystone, on the northwest corner of the Main St. and South Temple intersection. A squat, salmon-colored 19th-century obelisk cozies up to the Temple Square wall and bears the chiseled title Great Salt Lake Base and Meridian. Predating the term itself, this is ground zero, essentially 0 East and 0 South, as the streets South Temple and Main are the city's "zeroes." West Temple, then, is 100 West; State St. is 100 East; and North Temple is 100 North. Generally speaking, the numbering system subsequently adds another 100 for the streets bounding the area's large blocks, north, east, south, and west. Thus we next have 200 North, 200 South, etc. (However, in local parlance, they are often called Second North, Second South, and so on.) A marker notes that Brigham Young selected the temple site and meridian base on July 28, 1847—four days after he arrived in the Salt Lake Valley. A reminder of the elevation for those accustomed to walking and jogging closer to sea level: the site sits 4,327.27 feet above sea level. On the sidewalk nearby is the Old Folks Day marker, erected in 1936. It tells us a day was set aside in 1875 to honor all people age 70 and over. Of course, today many 70-plus people are likely to be out for a brisk walk in historic Salt Lake City. Nearby is the commanding Brigham Young Monument, but, trust us, we'll return to it later.

● Follow Temple Square's east wall north to the midblock reflective pool. You are on the Main Street Plaza, formerly a traffic-choked thoroughfare and now owned and maintained by the LDS Church as a walkway, garden, and gathering place. Explore. Sit. People-watch. Visitors often pause here. Around Christmastime, the plaza and Temple Square itself are ablaze with hundreds of thousands of festive lights. In spring, summer, and autumn the plaza and pool are a portrait-taking magnet for brides and their photographers and for passersby. The plaza is filled with garden spots and numerous plaques and statues, including vigorous figures of Joseph Smith, the founder and first prophet of the LDS Church, and Brigham Young, walking-cane in hand.

● The plaza pool's most prominent reflection, though, towers above: the many-turreted Salt Lake LDS Temple itself. Built of light gray, mica-speckled granite quarried in Little Cottonwood Canyon, about 20 miles to the valley's southeast, the neo-Gothic Salt Lake Temple is topped by a golden, trumpet-bearing angel. The temple took 40 years to build, finally receiving worshippers in 1893. Today, only Mormons deemed worthy by church leaders enter the temple, where important rites, such as baptisms and eternal marriages, are performed. Much of the garden around the temple is walled off or difficult to approach. Still, watch along the temple's tall east-side portals for even more formal postwedding photo ops starring brides, grooms, and extended families.

● Enter Temple Square proper through its iron east gate. You will find a display map of the entire LDS campus, a video screen, and, probably, the first paired missionary-guides, usually young women assigned here from around the world. Offering pleasant greetings, the guides are not here to proselytize per se, instead providing as little or as much information as you like. They, and others inside the square's South and North Visitor Centers, may offer to lead you on a leisurely tour of the grounds, which you can decline or which may be of interest, depending on your timetable. The walled and gated square is open daily, 9 a.m.–9 p.m. (If you are strolling outside during those hours, circle the block west to 50 N. West Temple and pick up directions for this walk from the Family History Library, noted below.) Between the temple and the South Visitor Center are more gardens and statuary, including the looming figures of Joseph Smith and his brother, Hyrum, who were murdered by a mob at a jail in Carthage, Illinois, in 1844.

● Proceed south, then immediately west, along the South Visitor Center. Step inside via the west entrance, if you wish, as the building features exhibits about LDS beliefs—plus restrooms and a respite from winter snow or summer heat. One display showcases a replica of the gold-leaf Angel Moroni, which graces spires of this and most other LDS temples around the world. Moroni is a key figure in Book of Mormon scripture and in the LDS belief in the restoration of the gospel that led to the church's founding in 1830. A recent addition to this visitor center is an intricate, to-scale model version of the Salt Lake Temple itself. Like a supersized dollhouse, one side is cut away to show what is inside the otherwise off-limits temple, complete with miniature murals, pews, and water fonts. The real thing rises majestically before you, just beyond the huge plate-glass window.

● Exit the South Visitor Center's west entrance to proceed deeper into south-central Temple Square, a forest of monuments, statues, and points of interest too many to enumerate. One prominent and unusual example is Seagull Monument. It is a memorial to birds believed to have saved pioneer crops by eating black crickets (today known as Mormon crickets) that were devastating the settlement's crops. The seagull is also Utah's state bird. Another evocative monument remembers impoverished

Salt Lake LDS Temple

pioneers who trudged across the plains and mountains to Salt Lake City pulling heavily laden handcarts.

- Moving on, in the square's southwest corner is the charming Assembly Hall, a traditional meetinghouse built in 1877 with granite left over from the temple construction. The building's truncated white spires, a marker informs us, were once chimneys.

- Besides its namesake, a famed centerpiece of Temple Square is the silver-domed Salt Lake Tabernacle, home of the Mormon Tabernacle Choir. An innovative architectural and acoustic feat in its time, the tabernacle, completed in 1867, seats 5,000 people and is generally open daily. Consider stepping inside door 11 to admire the tabernacle's pioneer handiwork and impressive 11,623-pipe organ. Again, interior tours are offered. For a pleasant pause, drop by the tabernacle for a half-hour organ recital, Monday–Saturday at noon and Sunday at 2 p.m. The public may also attend free choir rehearsals most Thursdays at 8 p.m. and the choir's long-running radio and TV program, *Music and the Spoken Word,* on Sunday at 9:30 a.m. (Please be seated by 9:15 for live performances.) Walkers can always set aside time later for the tours and concerts, or attend an event and continue the tour afterward.

- Near the tabernacle is the North Visitor Center. A quiet sanctuary (with public restrooms), it showcases detailed religious murals and artwork tied to the life, death, and resurrection of Jesus Christ; several video programs; and an 11-foot-tall white-marble replica of Danish sculptor Bertel Thorvaldsen's *Christus,* the resurrected Christ dramatically set among planets and stars depicted in a vaulting, painted background.

- Exit through the visitor center's south door, turn right, and follow the walkway toward the grounds' west gate. Just beyond you'll find the historic Nauvoo Bell Tower. Its plaques tell us the bronze bell was originally hung in the temple that LDS Church members built in Nauvoo, Illinois, in the 1840s. The Latter-day Saints removed the bell in 1846, doing so (according to a plaque) "when they were forced to leave Illinois because of persecution." Exit Temple Square via the west gate.

- Use the crosswalk to ford West Temple, which is blessed here with a traffic signal. Here are two more LDS buildings to tempt you. For many genealogists and family history enthusiasts, including those with no Mormon ties, the LDS Church's Family History Library is the reason to spend time in Salt Lake City. It houses the most extensive collection of genealogical records in the world. To the north is the Museum of Church History and Art, which features a collection of historic and contemporary LDS artifacts and art. Between the two buildings sits a restored log house dating to the pioneers' arrival in 1847. It was, notes an informational sign, originally the residence of Osmyn and Mary Deuel and Osmyn's brother, Amos, a family of blacksmiths and farmers.

- Heading north, cross North Temple and walk along the west side of the LDS Conference Center. The massive building actually rises from a deep setting, its comparatively low rooftop landscaped as a garden and arboretum. Completed in 2000 to host the LDS Church's semiannual general conference, as well as other church and community events, the facility houses a vast auditorium that seats 21,000 people, with a smaller theater on the side. Its granite face originated from the same quarry that produced stone for the Salt Lake Temple a century earlier. A waterfall cascades down the building's front, across from Temple Square.

- For our walk's sake, continue north along the conference center's west side and turn right on 200 North. Continue uphill eastward for one block (this route's most difficult section). A grove of trees grows on terraces along the conference center's northern exposure. The fancy home across Main St. and 200 North is the McCune Mansion, built in 1901. Turn right, to the south, at Main St. and stroll downhill. (Again, if you have time, free tours are available inside the conference center via door 1, as is access to the rooftop garden, which offers splendid views of Temple Square and downtown Salt Lake City.)

- At Main St. and North Temple, turn left and head east across Main. The LDS Church History Library, a 230,000-square-foot state-of-the-art facility, occupies the intersection's northeast corner. Free tours are available for this building, and the public is allowed to peruse many of its holdings.

- Turn right and cross North Temple. The elegant white Relief Society Building, built to house the LDS Church's women's organizations and completed in 1956, is on the opposite (southeast) corner, where one again enters the Main Street Plaza. Turn left before the reflecting pool and walk along the south side of the 28-story LDS Church Office Building. Free tours of the building's 26th-floor observation level are available during business hours and offer an unsurpassed bird's-eye view of all of Salt Lake City and its mountain-rimmed valley.

- Intersecting State St., turn left toward North Temple, then right (east) at the intersection, and cross busy State St. On the intersection's southeast corner is Brigham Young Historic Park, named for the Vermont native and pioneer leader. Markers

Back Story

Pioneer leader Brigham Young's presence and legacy can be found everywhere in Salt Lake City, from statuary to place names, especially in midtown, and in his home, the Beehive House. Mark Twain was but one of many visitors of note there, and Twain certainly left one of the funniest memories of a chat with the great colonizer in his Western memoir—part truth, part tall tale—*Roughing It.*

In the 1860s, Twain, then young Samuel Clemens of course, was en route to Nevada via stagecoach with his brother Orion, who was to be the secretary of the territory of Nevada, just to Utah's west. He found Young to be "a quiet, kindly, easy-mannered, dignified, self-possessed old gentleman of fifty-five or sixty and [he] had a gentle craft in his eye that probably belonged there." The humorist makes himself sound like a smart aleck, trying to "draw him out" regarding federal politics "and his high-handed attitude toward congress" (later, an apt description of Twain), to no avail. Young ignored him until the

visit's end, when "he put his hand on my head, beamed down at me in an admiring way, and said to my brother, 'Ah—your child, I presume? Boy or girl?'"

In her own reminiscence of life in the Beehive House as a child, *Brigham Young at Home*, Clarissa Young Spencer recalled visits by influential newspaperman Horace Greeley, who interviewed her father; British explorer Richard F. Burton, who wrote about his sojourn in the book *The City of the Saints;* Civil War General William Tecumseh Sherman; Schuyler Colfax, the powerful speaker of the U.S. House of Representatives; and famed actors and actresses of the day. Spencer was thrilled, though, to meet and dine with Tom Thumb, the tiny but renowned circus midget. In conversation, as Spencer tells it, Tom Thumb brought up a controversial subject. "'There is one thing I can't understand and that is this belief in polygamy.' Smiling down at him, Father answered very genially, 'I couldn't understand it either when I was your size.'"

note that this spot and much of what we've just visited were parts of his farm and orchards. Inside is a looping walkway, a water wheel powered by City Creek, and statues of pioneers tilling their fields. The park is particularly popular in summer, when chairs are set up and free concerts presented on Tuesday and Friday evenings.

- Exit the park and walk a half block south (left) down State St. Cross First Ave., turn left on the street's south side, and walk about 180 yards to find the gated Mormon Pioneer Memorial between sets of older houses and apartments. Enter this minipark, which pays homage to the sacrifice of more than 6,000 pioneers who died crossing the plains between 1847 and the completion of the Transcontinental Railroad in 1869. Monuments also review a few of their favorite songs (complete with bronzed sheet music). But this is also Brigham Young's family cemetery, where the Mormon leader was buried in 1877. Other stones mark the burials of a son and several of his wives.

- Upon leaving the small park, turn left and return down First Ave. to State St.; turn left (south) again, toward South Temple. You can't help but note the Eagle Gate spanning State St. This once marked the entrance to Brigham Young's estate. A plaque outlines the history of the gate and the creation of its magnificent eagle.

- Turn right at the intersection, crossing State St. On the corner stands the handsome, restored Beehive House, built of adobe and plaster in the early 1850s as Brigham Young's official residence. Atop the Greek Revival mansion's cupola is the namesake beehive (or "bee-hive," according to some signage)—still Utah's symbol. The Mormon beehive's call to industry, Mark Twain noted, "was simple, unostentatious, and fitted like a glove." After Brigham Young's death, the house and its adjoining offices continued to be the LDS Church headquarters and the residence of four succeeding LDS Church presidents. For a step back in time, consider taking a Beehive House tour, offered Monday through Saturday from 9 a.m. to 9 p.m.

- The Lion House, constructed next door in 1856, is another of Brigham Young's residences and home to many of his wives and children. Today it is a social center, hosting meetings and wedding parties, and offers a restaurant on the lower level, The Lion House Pantry. The wafting aromas of baking bread and roasting meats might be enough to draw you inside for a hearty meal.

- Next door to the west is the neoclassical-style, colonnaded Church Administration Building, completed in 1917. It includes the offices of the general authorities—the presiding leaders of the LDS Church—and is not open to the public.

- Just to the west, beyond more lovely campus gardens, stands the stately, century-old Joseph Smith Memorial Building, renamed and dedicated in 1988 to the founder of the LDS Church when it was converted into office and other multifunction spaces. For most of the 20th century, however, this was Hotel Utah, "the 'grand dame' of hotels in the Intermountain West," as one tour sign says. The 10-story structure—topped by another gargantuan beehive—was completed in 1911, its exterior gleaming with white-enameled brick and terra-cotta figures. Enter the building on South Temple via the revolving door to experience the warmth and rich décor of what once was Utah's premier hotel and social gathering place. Today it boasts a chapel, a gift shop, three restaurants (one at street level, two on the top floor), a 500-seat theater, a genealogy-oriented Family Search Center, public restrooms, and, of course, free tours.

● Return to the sidewalk, either on South Temple or the Main Street Plaza, to take in the route's final prize, the regal Brigham Young Monument. Until 1993, traffic rounded this monument, as it was in the center of the intersection. Today it rules the southern end of Main Street Plaza, Brother Brigham's arm outstretched toward his metropolitan legacy. Figures of a Native American and a mountain man bracket the towering pedestal, but a bronze placard clearly states that this monument was placed "in honor of Brigham Young and the Pioneers." In fact, a large plaque names the pioneers "who arrived in this valley, July 24, 1847," with a star signifying "those now living" (the monument was unveiled in 1897, the 50th anniversary of their arrival). The memorial notes: "The entire company and outfit consisted of 143 men, 3 women, 2 children, 70 wagons, 1 boat, 1 cannon, 93 horses, 52 mules, 66 oxen, 19 cows." Just to the west is Temple Square's southeastern corner, and you have returned to your starting point, Salt Lake City's meridian marker.

POINTS OF INTErEST (STArT TO FINISH)

Temple Square visittemplesquare.com, 15 E. South Temple, 801-240-1706

LDS Church History Museum lds.org/churchhistory/museum, 45 N. West Temple, 801-240-3310

LDS Conference Center lds.org/placestovisit/eng/visitors-centers/conference-center, northwest corner of North Temple and Main St., 801-240-0075

Beehive House lds.org, NW corner of South Temple and State St., 801-240-2681

The Lion House Pantry Restaurant templesquarehospitality.com/lionhouse, 63 E. South Temple, 801-539-3257

Joseph Smith Memorial Building templesquarehospitality.com/jsmb, 15 E. South Temple, 801-539-3130

route summary

1. Start at the northwest corner of the intersection of Main St. and South Temple, which is the southeast corner of Temple Square.

2. Walk north a half block to 50 N. Main St., touring Main Street Plaza; then enter Temple Square's east gate.

3. Explore Temple Square, its monuments and open buildings (the South and North Visitor Centers, Assembly Hall, the Salt Lake Tabernacle), and exit the west gate at 50 N. West Temple.

4. Cross West Temple at the midblock signal, site of the Family History Library and Museum of Church History and Art; then turn right up West Temple to North Temple.

5. Cross North Temple and walk north to 200 North along the west side of the LDS Conference Center.

6. Turn right (east) on 200 North and continue uphill to Main St.

7. Turn right again (south) on Main St. to North Temple, along the conference center's east side.

8. Cross Main St. (the LDS Church History Library is ahead) and turn right to cross North Temple.

9. Follow the Main Street Plaza past the Relief Society Building and turn east at midblock and pass the Church Office Building.

10. At State St., turn left to North Temple.

11. Go left across North Temple to Brigham Young Historical Park.

12. Upon leaving the park, turn left and walk down State St. a half block to First Ave.

13. Turn left on the south side of First Ave., continuing about 180 yards to the Mormon Pioneer Memorial.

14. Upon leaving the park, turn left, return (west), and turn left on State St., continuing south to the Eagle Gate.

15. Turn left at South Temple and cross State St. to Brigham Young's Beehive House.

16. Here in sequence you will walk west along South Temple, passing (or visiting) the Beehive House, the LDS Church Administration Building, the Joseph Smith Memorial Building, and the Brigham Young Monument, returning to the tour's starting point.

connecting the walks

Connect with Walk 7, Memory Grove/City Creek Canyon, at State St. and North Temple.

Connect with Walk 9, East South Temple, at State St. and South Temple.

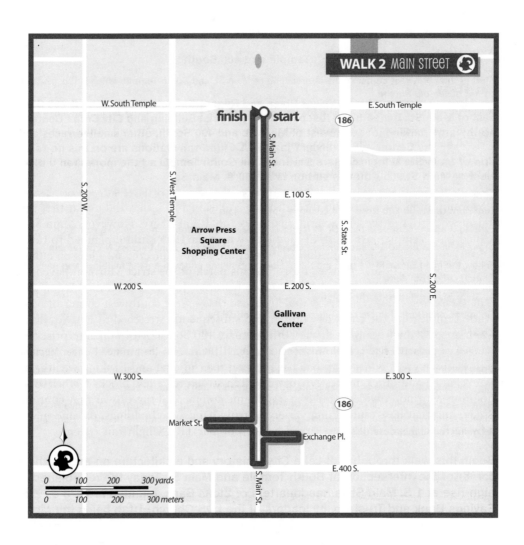

W. South Temple

E. South Temple

finish   start

186

S. Main St.

S. West Temple

S. 200 W.

E. 100 S.

S. State St.

**Arrow Press
Square
Shopping Center**

W. 200 S.

E. 200 S.

S. 200 E.

**Gallivan
Center**

W. 300 S.

E. 300 S.

186

Market St.

Exchange Pl.

E. 400 S.

S. Main St.

0   100   200   300 yards
0   100   200   300 meters

2 Main Street: a DOWNTOWN TUG-OF-war

BOUNDARIES: **Main St., between South Temple and 400 South**
DISTANCE: **1.25 miles**
DIFFICULTY: **Easy**
PARKING: **Metered street parking; Walker Plaza and Regent St. parking terraces off 200 South east of Main St.; beneath the Joseph Smith Memorial Building and City Creek Center on the north; large parking lot southwest of Main St. and 400 South; other small terraces and lots**
PUBLIC TRANSIT: **City Center and Gallivan Plaza TRAX light-rail stations are on this no-fare portion of Main St.; Temple Square Station is on South Temple a little more than a block west of Main St.; courthouse station is at 450 S. Main St.**

When Mormon pioneers arrived in the Salt Lake Valley in 1847, they did not at first provide for a business district in their new, grid-based Great Salt Lake City. However, Main St., originally called East Temple, just south of the block where the LDS faithful planned to raise their grand new temple, soon began to fulfill that function. Stores squeezed into lots on either side of the street—as did saloons. By the late 1850s this patch of the strict Mormon haven was known with a wink as Whiskey St., according to historian John S. McCormick's *Salt Lake City: The Gathering Place*. The first Council House rose on the southwest corner of Main St. and South Temple, and the city's downtown hub subsequently stretched to 200 South, then 300 South and, by the beginning of the 20th century, 400 South. Mormon enterprises, notably Zion's Cooperative Mercantile Institution (ZCMI), came to dominate the northern section of this downtown core. Non-Mormons began using their mining and banking wealth to build a stock exchange and other impressive metropolitan structures a few blocks farther south. The Mormon/non-Mormon divide resulted in a dynamic commercial tug-of-war that continues to this day, and that has resulted in a variety of truly handsome buildings, old and new, all linked by active city sidewalks and served by the popular TRAX light-rail system.

● **Begin this walk through Salt Lake City's history and architecture on the southeast corner of the intersection of South Temple and Main St. Today the refurbished high-rise at 1 S. Main St. is headquarters of Zions Bank, founded in 1873 as Zion's Savings Bank and Trust Co. by leaders of the LDS Church—Utah being the Mormon Zion, their promised land. Although it is now Zions Bancorporation, a financial institution with branches in 10 Western states, many Utahns still think of it as Zions**

First National Bank, which it was through most of a century. Not that long ago, this modest skyscraper was sheathed in distinctive copper panels and was home to the Kennecott Copper Corp., now part of the international Rio Tinto mining conglomerate.

● Walk south along Main St.'s east side and you enter the massive City Creek Center. Old Main St. is the spine of this new open-air mall, which blankets almost 20 acres. The east and west sides of Main St. and of City Creek Center are linked by a midblock bridge suspended over the busy thoroughfare and TRAX lines, near the City Center TRAX station. The redevelopment project has taken the bridal adage of "something old, something new" to heart. A prime example: the three-story, cast-iron ZCMI façade, an intricate bit of heavy-metal lacework saved and restored to its historic place as the entry to Macy's department store. The façade's pillars and arches first fronted ZCMI in 1876. Long advertised as America's first department store, ZCMI was founded in 1868 as a multipronged enterprise to counter the more expensive stores of incoming non-Mormon merchants. The cast-iron façade was expanded in 1880 and 1901 and restored and replaced when ZCMI became part of a new mall in the 1970s. ZCMI was purchased by the May Co. in 1999. The company subsequently added and expanded the historic Macy's chain, which came to include this location. The façade, which is on the National Register of Historic Places, was again dismantled for the City Creek Center project, to be resurrected once again as the antique face of a new Macy's.

● Continue toward 100 South, and just before the corner you will meet the Deseret Building, at 79 S. Main St. A bank has been here since the 1850s, one placard notes, making it the oldest continuously operated banking site in Utah. Pioneer-era Hooper & Eldredge bank was succeeded in 1871 by the Bank of Deseret, headed by none other than Brigham Young, and in 1872 by the nationally chartered Deseret National Bank. The classic, columnlike tower now on the corner was built in 1919 with, as the Utah Heritage Foundation describes it, a three-story pedestal decorated with Indian heads and bison, an eight-story shaft, and an ornate three-story capital. Deseret National merged with Security National Bank in 1932 to form First Security Bank, long one of the region's financial heavyweights. Wells Fargo absorbed First Security into its empire in 2000.

● Cross 100 South to midblock. You've passed buildings of now-defunct 20th-century banks and savings-and-loan institutions. The locations have served a variety of purposes over the decades, from department stores (including the once mighty Montgomery Ward) to jewelry and clothing outlets. At 143 S. Main St. stands a brown-brick tower with a terra-cotta cornice, 1924's Ezra Thompson/Salt Lake Tribune Building. Even earlier, this was the site of a Pony Express office, as two different markers point out. One plaque, topped by a dashing man and horse, is inset into the building's entryway; another is a freestanding granite-and-bronze monument toward the nearby curb. Both tell of the brief (1860–1861) but legendary experiment in which lone riders carrying mail packets skedaddled between St. Joseph, Missouri, and Sacramento, California. Yet another plaque inset into the building commemorates the long history of *The Salt Lake Tribune*, established in 1870, as does a tour-stop marker bearing the number 19. The latter is one of many you'll see that were placed throughout the downtown area by the Utah Heritage Foundation before the 2002 Winter Olympic Games, hosted by Salt Lake City. The *Tribune*, once the community's non-Mormon bastion, remains Utah's largest-circulation newspaper but has moved to new quarters in the Gateway complex on the west side of downtown.

● As you resume your stroll south, you'll pass the former First National Bank Building, built in 1873, which features what is believed to be the oldest cast-iron façade in the West. Next is the U-shaped Salt Lake Herald Building, once home to another of the city's many early newspapers. Like the building's construction date (1905), the journal's name remains a prominent part of the high tin cornice, although the newspaper moved out in 1913. Lamb's Grill Cafe, one of downtown's iconic restaurants and a fabled meeting place for the city's power brokers, has occupied the ground floor since 1919. If you enjoy traditional American fare with ambience, Lamb's is a flavorful stop for

Daft Block

breakfast, lunch, or dinner. Walking inside is like a step back in time, with a long vintage dining counter, small side booths with wooden seat backs, linen-covered tables, and a big back room for larger parties.

- After passing several budding eateries, you will reach the northeast corner of Main St. and 200 South. The Walker Bank Building looms 16 stories overhead. Completed in 1912, this was at the time the tallest building between Denver and the West Coast. As the Utah Heritage Foundation has phrased it, the early skyscraper proved "a source of much pride to Salt Lake City." Today Far West Bank occupies part of the building. The top two stories are classically ornamented. A smaller three-story observatory sits atop the tall building—itself crowned with eagles and a 64-foot lighted weather tower that bears the structure's current name, Walker Center. Beginning in the 1950s, a metal tower with the bank's name beamed a weather forecast at night, but it was taken down in the 1980s. Restored in 2008, the landmark sign again offers a color-coded forecast: blue for clear skies, flashing blue for cloudy skies, red for rain, and flashing red for snow.

- Cross 200 South to the 24-story One Utah Center. The modern pink-granite and glass skyscaper is topped by a copper pyramid that, as part of the city's skyline, gleams at night like a multifaceted jewel. Glance down on the corner sidewalk and you'll notice a colorful series of artwork squares. The large, color-splashed tiles are inlaid with glass and etched photographs of people and scenes from Utah's history, such as the joining of the Transcontinental Railroad, which occurred in Utah in 1869. South and east of the center is Gallivan Plaza, a midcity park where people can walk, sit, and eat. The plaza hosts midday and evening concerts in the summer.

- Continue beyond Gallivan Plaza's Main St. entry. In mid–Main St. to the right is a busy TRAX station sharing the plaza's name. To the south, occupying the northeast corner of 300 South and Main St., is the Wells Fargo Center. Also a 24-story skyscraper, it was built in 1998 as the national headquarters of American Stores. CBS television affiliate KUTV Channel 2 broadcasts from the street level. A large-screen TV is on the building's northwest corner above the sidewalk, and newscasters, predominately members of the weather team, often report outside from Main St. or the Gallivan Center. So be forewarned: You might be on the news as you walk by.

● Cross 300 South and you have entered Main St.'s century-old non-Mormon downtown. Magnates such as Samuel Newhouse and Orange J. Salisbury had their hearts set on shifting Salt Lake City's commercial hub south, away from the Mormon-dominated sector on north Main St. In sequence along this block's east side are historic buildings of varied heights built by developers with that mindset. Not all of the developers were men: The Judge Building, on the intersection's southeast corner, was built by business-savvy widow and philanthropist Mary Judge, a marker says. After the early death of her wealthy husband John, she multiplied her fortune with investments in local real estate and Nevada mines. Salisbury built the Felt Building, which showcases the state's first terra-cotta façade, including classic Greek cameos beneath a pale leaf pattern. Another bevy of small eateries can be found along this block.

● At midblock, 350 S. Main St., your walk intersects Exchange Place—Samuel Newhouse's would-be Wall Street West. On the Main St. corners, Newhouse built the fraternal-twin stone-and-brick Boston and Newhouse Buildings between 1907 and 1909. Considered Utah's first true skyscrapers, each has 11 stories, and both have a three-part design: main floor, a vertical office shaft in the center, and an elaborate cornice. Newhouse hired legendary Chicago–New York architect Henry Ives Cobb to design the structures. The Boston is graced with a series of floral-wrapped stone shields, as well as lions near the roof. It is named after Newhouse's Boston Consolidated Copper and Gold Mining Co., which harvested metals in Bingham Canyon on the valley's west side. The Newhouse, of course, he named after himself. Look up: Petrified cornucopias and flowers line the exterior, and the huge, curly furred head of a bison hovers above Main St.

● Detour briefly a half block east into Exchange Place, the core of this mini Wall Street. A small plaza at the Main St. corner blocks through-traffic. Newhouse contributed land on Exchange Place for two substantial buildings that non-Mormon entrepreneurs erected in the early 1900s. At 39 Exchange Place, on the street's north side, is the colonnaded Salt Lake Stock and Mining Exchange, built in 1908. Built to raise capital for Utah's early mines, it remained a hotbed of stock sales through eras such as the 1950s uranium boom and the rise of penny stocks. Today lawyers and architects have offices in the venerable financial center. Across the way, at 32 Exchange Place, is one of Salt Lake City's most beautiful—and least visible—architectural showpieces, the secluded Commercial Club. Erected in 1909, the building's brickwork boasts polychromatic terra-cotta panels with bright mosaics. Inside the luxurious Commercial Club—apparently part early Chamber of Commerce, part metropolitan men's club—were game and banquet rooms and a basement swimming pool.

- Return west to Main St. and turn south toward the northeast corner of Main St. and 400 South. Here yet another mining magnate, John Daly, built the New Grand Hotel in 1910. The hotel's deep-red brick is inlaid with colorful tiles, arranged in horizontal designs between floors.

- Turn right at 400 South and cross to Main St.'s west side. Fierce-looking eagles guard a double staircase at 350 S. Main St. Deeply incised beyond the raptors, block letters confirm that this magisterial 1905 building, later enlarged and sheathed in granite, is firmly planted in the United States of America. At first it housed Salt Lake City's main U.S. post office and other government functions, including the federal court. Today it is strictly the Frank E. Moss Federal Courthouse, named for a late senator. True to the cultural tug-of-war, the location of this building was a matter of contention after Utah finally became a state in 1896. The LDS Church offered a site across from Temple Square, historians say. The non-Mormon businessmen of growing, turn-of-the-century south Main St. objected—and won this downtown skirmish.

- Continue to Market St. (340 S. Main St.), north of the courthouse, and turn left, strolling west about a quarter block. This will give you a good view, across the narrow midblock alley, of two more historic buildings on the street's north side. On the left is the New Yorker. To its right is a building with an odd tale: Odd Fellows Hall. Cross the street for a closer look—or a meal—if you'd like. Until recently, the ornate 1891 brick Odd Fellows Hall would have been behind you, on Market St.'s south side. To allow for courthouse expansion, the antiquated building was shored up, lifted, and moved across the street as part of a preservation effort. The International Order of Odd Fellows (IOOF) was one of numerous secret social, charitable, and fraternal societies that emerged in 19th-century America to help members and their families in times of illness and death—an early form of insurance well before Medicare and Medicaid. The New Yorker, recently painted a light green, was once the comfortable New York Hotel, a high-tech inn when it was built in 1906 by Orange J. Salisbury: It had electric lights and steam heat in every room. In 1978 Gastronomy Inc. pioneered the restoration and rejuvenation of historic buildings in Salt Lake City when it opened the New Yorker on the lower level, which has become a celebrated restaurant. The atmospheric Market Street Grill and Oyster Bar attract patrons salivating for quality seafood and steak at the sidewalk level.

● Return east to Main St. and turn left at The Melting Pot, a restaurant specializing in fondue dishes, walking north to 300 South. The brick-and-glass tower on the inter-section's southwest corner, at 310 S. Main St., is the modern headquarters of the J.C. Penney department store chain. Cross 300 South—which is also called Broadway here in the city center—to the Clift Building, on the northwest corner. Highly decorative and faced with terra-cotta, it was built by widow and businesswoman Virtue Clift in 1920 in honor of her late husband, Francis. Continue north to the Keith Building, long the home of Sam Weller's Bookstore, which recently moved to nearby Trolley Square. The building that bears his name was commissioned by mining magnate-merchant David Keith, whose wealth came from the silver mines of Park City, Utah.

● North of the Keith are several small buildings, or blocks, in the terminology of a cen-tury ago. They include the classically ornate Lollin Block and the carved-stone and cast-iron Karrick Block, designed by Richard Kletting, best known as the architect of the Utah State Capitol. The new granite-and-glass high-rise at 222 S. Main St. has taken its location to heart: Called 222 Main, it has been awarded gold certification by the group Leadership in Energy and Environmental Design (LEED). To its north is the lanky, 13-story Continental Bank Building, at 208 S. Main St. Completed in 1924, the very vertical skyscraper was refurbished in 1999 to become the deluxe Hotel Monaco, with the swanky and much-praised Bambara Restaurant at street level.

● Cross 200 South and proceed past a collection of small buildings and the entry to the vacant Utah Theater (once one of downtown's finest movie houses) to the richly decorated Kearns Building, at 136 S. Main St. This Sullivan-esque high-rise, built in 1911, proves that not all of the buildings raised by non-Mormon magnates are to downtown's south. This is a monument to one of Utah's richest and most prominent men, Thomas Kearns. A wag once pegged it the state's real capitol. Kearns arrived in Utah penniless, according to the Utah Heritage Foundation, but with friend and partner David Keith hit it big in the silver mines of Park City. Kearns became a U.S. senator and part owner of *The Salt Lake Tribune.* The female faces in the chorus line overhead are believed to resemble his daughter, Helen. The Kearns Building continues to be an important downtown office building. At street level is an Italian restaurant, Michelangelo's on Main.

● Continuing north, the ornate brick Daft Block, with its projecting bay window, seems tiny next to the hulking Kearns Building. Built, like a few others along Main, by a miner's widow, it is one of the city's oldest structures, dating to 1889. As a brightly painted sign on the north side still reminds us, this was long the home of Daynes Jewelry, a company founded by a pioneer watchmaker. The Daft now offers a draft; it houses the retro-modern Beehive Pub. But on the southwest corner of Main St. and 100 South is Salt Lake City's real survivor. This was the Eagle Emporium when merchant William Jennings built it in 1864. It is downtown's only pioneer-era commercial building that predates the arrival of the Transcontinental Railroad in 1869. Originally possessing a sandstone façade, it was given a gleaming terra-cotta veneer in 1916. The emporium was the first home of ZCMI in 1868, became a bank in 1890, and has long been an office of Zions First National Bank (Zion Bank), as it says near the rooftop. Step inside for a peek at how banking used to be done, amid woodwork, at teller's cages, and beneath portraits of the powerful and distinguished. The corner also hosts an antique standing clock, also known as street furniture. Erected in 1873 and still (usually) keeping time, it was powered at first by a water wheel . . . somehow.

● Cross 100 South to the north. Though not so imposing today, the seven-story McCornick Block on the intersection's northwest corner towered over its squat two- to four-story neighbors when it went up in 1893. It even had elevators! An addition was made on the north side in 1908; then the McIntyre Building next door, built in 1898 at 68 S. Main St., stretched to the sky yet another story. The new but varied buildings farther along the block are part of downtown's new City Creek Center development, with a sky bridge linking Main St.'s western and eastern sides. End your walk through history at the intersection with South Temple. The 19-story Gateway Tower rises on this prime spot today, but Salt Lake City's original Council House stood here from 1850 to 1883, when a fire and explosion gutted Utah's first public building and occasional territorial statehouse.

POINTS OF INTEREST (START TO FINISH)

ZCMI façade and City Creek Center about 30 S. Main St.

Pony Express site 143 S. Main St.

Herald Building and Lamb's Grill Cafe lambsgrill.com, 169 S. Main St., 801-364-7166

Exchange Place, Boston and **Newhouse Buildings** 350 S. Main St.

Frank E. Moss Federal Courthouse/former U.S. Post Office 350 S. Main St.

New Yorker gastronomyinc.com, 60 W. Market St., 801-363-0166

Market Street Grill gastronomyinc.com, 48 W. Market St., 801-322-4668

The Melting Pot meltingpot.com, 340 S. Main St., 801-521-6358

Keith Building 254 S. Main St.

Hotel Monaco and Bambara Restaurant bambara-slc.com, 202 S. Main St., 801-363-5454

Kearns Building and Michelangelo's on Main 132 S. Main St., 801-532-0500

Beehive Pub 128 S. Main St., 801-364-4268

route summary

1. Start at the southeast corner of South Temple and Main St.
2. Walk south on Main St., crossing 100 South, 200 South, and 300 South.
3. Turn left and walk east a half block into Exchange Place (350 S. Main St.).
4. Return west to Main St.
5. Turn left and continue south to 400 South.
6. Cross Main St. at 400 South.
7. Turn right and continue north along Main St. to Market Place (340 S. Main St.).
8. Turn left and walk west a half block into Market Place.
9. Return east to Main St.
10. Turn left and walk north on Main St., crossing 300 South, 200 South, and 100 South.
11. Complete the route at the intersection of Main St. and South Temple.

CONNECTING THE WALKS

Since Main St. is downtown Salt Lake City's central north-south artery, this walk links to several other walk options. The Temple Square campus and its Main Street Plaza are at the top of midtown Main St., where this walk begins. The City Creek Center area is sliced in half by Main St. The south downtown walk crosses a Main St. "T" at 400 South.

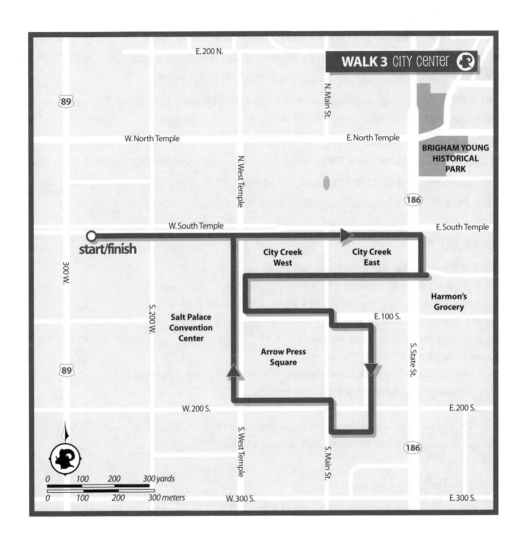

E. 200 N.

89

W. North Temple

N. Main St.

E. North Temple

BRIGHAM YOUNG HISTORICAL PARK

N. West Temple

186

W. South Temple

E. South Temple

start/finish

300 W.

S. 200 W.

City Creek West

City Creek East

Harmon's Grocery

Salt Palace Convention Center

S. West Temple

Arrow Press Square

E. 100 S.

S. State St.

89

W. 200 S.

S. Main St.

E. 200 S.

186

| 0 | 100 | 200 | 300 yards |
| 0 | 100 | 200 | 300 meters |

W. 300 S.

E. 300 S.

3 CITY CENTER: "GREAT" SALT LAKE CITY

BOUNDARIES: South Temple, State St., 250 South, and West Temple
DISTANCE: 2.5 miles
DIFFICULTY: Easy
PARKING: Curbside metered parking and several parking lots and terraces, including a new 5,000-spot underground parking area at City Creek Center, at 50 N. West Temple, at the Joseph Smith Memorial Building on South Temple, and at the Walker Center and Regent St. terraces accessed via 200 South, among others.
PUBLIC TRANSIT: Utah Transit Authority's TRAX light-rail runs along Main St., and thus through the middle of City Creek Center, with stops at 250 S. Main St. (Gallivan Center Station) and 50 S. Main St. (City Center Station). It turns on South Temple, with a stop near Abravanel Hall and Temple Square (132 W. South Temple, Temple Square Station). Numerous bus routes ply State St. and 200 South, in particular. The city's mid-downtown area, and to the State Capitol, is a limited Free Fare Zone for both buses and TRAX.

If metropolitan centers were a reality TV topic, Salt Lake City's heart would have just been the subject of *Extreme Downtown Makeover*. In fact, the show is still under way, and the world-class City Creek Center open-air complex is a major reason why. Rising against all odds during a worldwide recession, the $2 billion resurrection opened south of the Temple Square campus in March 2012. Named for the snow-fed, year-round stream so vital to the pioneers of 1847 and beyond, the retail center is eminently walkable and sustainably designed, an urban mix of shops, restaurants, apartments, and condominiums. And for visitors, it has a customer service and concierge counter.

This is the historic core of what was originally "Great Salt Lake City." (Despite the lake's proximity, the hyperbolic-seeming "Great" was gradually dropped in the 1850s.) The mall's builders and managers, including the LDS Church, seem to have focused on that ideal when they opted to demolish two monolithic midtown malls in 2006 and start anew. Despite the newness, the surrounding area—much of it part of this walk—is chockablock with history, from old skyscrapers to hotels, office towers, and arts and convention complexes of various eras. These include the Calvin L. Rampton Salt Palace Convention Center; the Salt Lake Art Center; Abravanel Hall (home of the Utah Symphony); the restored and expanded century-old Capitol Theatre, a showplace for Utah Opera and Broadway-style productions; art galleries; restaurants; and more.

City Creek Center pays homage, of sorts, to the pioneering city's age. Old and new seamlessly mingle. Where two blocky, Kremlin-walled retail behemoths (Crossroads Mall and the ZCMI Center) stood until 2006, individual buildings now grace the skyline. Many edifices are partly brick, not simply glass and steel, with fresh angles and an old-new look (Art Deco, anyone?). Anchored by Nordstrom and Macy's department stores, the 20-acre complex hosts more than 100 stores and restaurants; has an arched, retractable roof for when the weather turns nasty; and sports statuary, Las Vegas–style dancing fountains, a trout pond, and a manicured stream (bits of City Creek!). The project galvanized construction nearby as well, as the city continues to add even more new stores, housing, and office buildings.

And although outlets and restaurants may be closed in the wee hours, privately owned City Creek Center, like the surrounding downtown, is intended to be a strolling and window-shopping destination most hours of the day and night, open from 6:30 a.m. to midnight, seven days a week, year-round, though stores and the food court are closed on Sundays.

- **Begin your downtown business district walk at the southwest corner of South Temple and West Temple. At 123 W. South Temple is Abravanel Hall, distinguished outwardly by its triangular brick corner and massive pane-glass front. This is the home of the Utah Symphony. When the light is right, one can discern abstract dopplegangers of Temple Square and other nearby buildings in its reflective glass. A twisty Dale Chihuly blown-glass artwork swirls just inside. Lauded for its acoustics, the facility opened in 1979 and can seat more than 2,800 concert-goers.**

- **Walk east to the corner of West Temple and South Temple. Cross to the southeast corner and proceed along the south side of South Temple. On the north side is Temple Square. Almost the entire block to your right is occupied by City Creek Center West. On the intersection's southeast corner towers The Promontory, a 30-story, 370-foot-tall residential skyscraper. This is the tallest structure in the new mixed-use mall, boasting 344,000 square feet of living space. It offers residents stunning views of the Salt Lake Valley in every direction—especially the higher you go. The century-old haberdashery Utah Woolen Mills, at 59 W. South Temple, remained open for business during City Creek's multiblock renovation. Deseret Book, an LDS Church–owned publisher and bookstore chain, maintains its headquarters and flagship store here, as well. The twin, 10-story Richards Court towers are midblock at 45 and 55 W. South Temple. The Blue Lemon restaurant is on the ground floor of Richards Court West.**

Long ago, north-south Richards St. divided the block here, as embedded markers note. Richards St. has been reborn, in a way, offering street-level access to City Creek Center's interior. Continue walking east to Main St., toward Gateway Tower West, an office tower. Hagermann's Bakehouse Café entices passersby on the ground floor.

● At Main St., cross east, over the TRAX light-rail line, and continue along South Temple. Most of the standard 10-acre city block to your right is the new City Creek Center East. Pass the Zions Bank Building and you will note another street-level entrance to the interior of the shopping and dining complex. Next is the Eagle Gate Plaza and Tower, an office complex that connects to City Creek Center.

● Cross State St. to the east and then turn right (south). Historic Alta Club, founded by mining and business entrepreneurs in the 19th century, is on the corner. Just to its south is the mansionlike flagship store of Salt Lake–based jeweler O. C. Tanner, at 15 S. State St. The handsome building, on the National Register of Historic Places, was originally Salt Lake City's Main Library when it opened in 1904. After the library moved to more spacious quarters nearby, it served as home of Hansen Planetarium from the mid-1960s to 2003. Visitors are welcome to step into the elegantly remodeled building, named America's coolest store by a national retail magazine.

● At midblock to the south, beyond the historic brick Belvedere apartment turned condo tower, is Social Hall Ave., so named because the pioneer community's adobe Social Hall stood here, beginning in 1852. A bronze plaque beside the busy sidewalk offers passersby an image of the vanished amusement hall, and a glass-and-metal structure mimics its placement. This building is now the

A 100 South brownstone

entrance to a subterranean crossing beneath State St. to City Creek Center. The lower level is also a museum. Sections of the Social Hall's sandstone foundations, discovered here years ago, are on display, and illustrated wall panels tell the tale of the hall, a popular place for dances and small theatrical events. Displays showcase archaeological artifacts and period costumes. If the museum entry is closed, cross State St. at the intersection either to the north or to the south (South Temple or 100 South) to make your way to the new crux of it all: City Creek Center. *Note:* An unusual, new multistory Harmon's grocery store sits beyond Social Hall Ave., at 100 S. State St. Another major pioneer-era gathering place, the Salt Lake Theatre, once stood across the way; the spot is now marked by an impressive bronze wall placard.

● Using the Social Hall escalators or stairways, make your way west underground to City Creek Center. At a junction, turn right into the spacious, midblock food court, which opened in 2010 and continues to expand. Nearby, to the left of this entry, is a new indoor, dinosaur-themed playground, sitting, and eating area for children and their parents. The court's eateries include the usual suspects, from McDonald's to Subway, as well as ethnic cuisines, from Chinese and Japanese to Italian and Mexican, including A Taste of Red Iguana, a mall presence for local favorite Red Iguana.

● Exit the food court, walking west into the central plaza. An 18-foot-high landscaped waterfall feeds into City Creek Center's namesake streamlet, which, with human intervention, courses thither and yon through the modern dining, retail, and housing complex. A water motif decorates many walls and walkways and includes a flowing sculpture, *Stream,* crowded with images of gulls, a bear, an elk, otters, and topped by a swooping eagle. A large Cheesecake Factory Restaurant occupies a strategic location on the plaza's south end. A seasonal fire pit might be blazing on the second level to the north. Glance down to the main level's pavement stones and you'll occasionally catch sight of the incised prints of the Mountain West's wild creatures—perhaps a mountain lion, a bear, or a mule deer. Macy's, one of the center's anchor stores, has entrances on levels to the northwest. Need help or guidance? Just outside Macy's central main-level entrance is a customer service/concierge center. This is an excellent place to grab a brochure that includes a map and directory of City Creek Center. Informational screens here note airline departure times, offer ski reports, and present local travel advice. Near the information desk is an unusual mall feature: a "stream" and pond alive with darting trout.

- From the central plaza, make your way upstairs by escalator or elevator to the second level's store-lined walkway, over the lower sidewalks and pools. Above the plaza, turn right to walk west through the middle of City Creek. Modern urban views abound: office and apartment buildings, a busy retail scene, and "clamshell" arches with a secret. If the weather turns, the archways can, in about four minutes, pretty much silently turn this open-air pedestrian mall into a glass-enclosed one, or vice versa. Principal walkways are also heated by underground pipes in winter to prevent snow or ice buildup, and are cooled in summer by cold water percolating underfoot.

- At Main St. a sky bridge sprinkled with cut-glass leafy patterns spans the people, TRAX line, and traffic below. Outstanding cityscapes unfold to the south and north. Inset underfoot in the skywalk's center is a cast-metal map of Salt Lake City, circa 1871. And the skyway leads to the second level of City Creek Center West.

- The street- and second-level shops continue into the midst of this western block, with an open-to-the-sky circular plaza at its center. Descend via any of the escalators, stairways, or elevators to Richards Court—this was once Richards St.—which includes playful, squirting fountains (with names such as "Transcend" and "Engage") that rival many a Las Vegas water feature. Other fountains and streams align with Richards St. to the north and south; one called "Flutter" creates fanciful bubblelike flowing domes. Seating is plentiful for patrons in need of a restful moment—or a little people- or water-watching. Apartment and condominium residences, including the skyscraping Promontory to the northwest, overlook everything. Upscale outlets like Tiffany & Co., Rolex, and Swarovski occupy locations on the first and second levels. Nordstrom, on the fountain plaza's west side, is the multilevel anchor store of City Creek Center West. Stroll through Nordstrom to its street entrance on West Temple, which is colorfully illuminated at night.

- Exit Nordstrom and City Creek Center onto West Temple and turn left, walking south. The Salt Palace Convention Center is across the street. Pass the Marriott Hotel, cross 100 South, and turn left (east) on 100 South. A variety of restaurants and galleries line the street's south side, including Naked Fish Bistro; Utah Artist Hands gallery, which specializes in Utah-made crafts, paintings, and photography; and Caffé Molise. On the Main St. intersection's southeast corner, beside a historic store turned bank, is an antique street clock that dates back to 1873 and came to Utah in a wagon. (Find more about downtown Main St.'s history in Walk 2.)

- Cross Main St. to its southeast corner, continuing east. The 14-story Deseret Building, built in 1919 as a bank and narrowly saved from demolition in 2006, is across the way, on the interchange's northeast corner. On the south side of 100 South you'll pass a large building that has variously served as a department store (Montgomery Ward) and a bank; a historic sandstone-brownstone reminiscent of New York City; and, at midblock Regent St., a modern office building that formerly housed the *Deseret News,* Utah's oldest business. Just to the north, of course, are many of Utah's newest enterprises, part of the expansive City Creek Center downtown rejuvenation.

- At Regent St., turn right and head south. Short, north-south Regent St. boasted one of Salt Lake's first paved roads. Historians say this is because this was the city's red-light district at the turn of the 20th century. Regent St. hosted a number of brothels, and patrons didn't like coating their footwear with street mud or clay, for obvious reasons. More recently Regent St. bustled as the city's newspaper-publishing center. The presses and offices of both daily newspapers, *The Salt Lake Tribune* and the *Deseret News,* were here, or nearby, until editorial and printing operations recently moved away.

- At 200 South, which is graced with a flashing midblock pedestrian crossing for safety, head south to the Gallivan Center, a musical-cultural gathering place and park. Like other downtown locales, this plaza was renovated and reopened in late 2011. The new copper-faced building on the plaza's north side houses reception and meeting halls, restrooms, Patterson's Pub, and lockers for those using the park's expanded ice rink in winter. Meander through its sitting areas, urban art, and reminders of the 2002 Winter Olympic Games. An eye-catching mirrored tower topped by a sandstone boulder is just one of the plaza's artworks. It is *Asteroid Landed Softly,* a multicultural sundial created by Kazuo Matsubayashi. The park's grassy amphitheater and stage are popular concert and festival sites much of the year. Weather permitting, a fountain with curtains of water splashes west of the stage. Eventually turn west to a Main St. exit just south of pyramid-topped Utah One Center and north of the 24-story Wells Fargo Building, also home of KUTV, a local CBS TV station that often uses the handy outdoor Gallivan Center venues next door.

● You are at about 250 S. Main St. The UTA TRAX light-rail line employs a midstreet island as the Gallivan Center Station. Turn right and walk north on Main St. to 200 South (a half-block repeat of Walk 2) and cross to the north side. On the intersection's northeast corner, turn left to cross Main St., heading west along 200 South's north side, past a bank, a delicatessen, and other shops. At 50 W. 200 South is the lavishly decorated Art Deco Capitol Theatre. Built in 1913 as a vaudeville venue, today it is an arts haven, a 1,750-seat showplace for plays, musicals, and the Utah Opera, affiliated with the Utah Symphony. Across the street are an Olive Garden restaurant and two hotels (a Shilo Inn and a Hilton), as well as a bevy of restaurants associated with them. *Note:* More dining options are arrayed along nearby Pierpont Ave., a half block to the southwest.

● Upon reaching West Temple, cross to its west side and turn right, walking north along West Temple. On this block, and parts of others, sprawls the Calvin L. Rampton Salt Palace Convention Center, named for a popular three-term governor of the 1960s and '70s. Opened in the early 1990s, this version of the Salt Palace (other facilities have shared that name, including a predecessor on this site) encompasses some 675,000 square feet of exhibit and convention space and meeting rooms. Water features and decorative windmills lead to a signature glass-and-steel cylinder that marks the center's main entrance. To the north of this entry is the information office and gift shop of the Salt Lake Convention and Visitors Bureau, also known online as Visit Salt Lake. Step inside—you'll discover brochures and details about destinations and things to do in Salt Lake City and throughout Utah. Also on the complex's north side, at 20 S. West Temple, is the Salt Lake Art Center, a venue for contemporary visual arts, exhibits, workshops, a gift shop, and special events.

● Stroll farther along West Temple, toward the corner of South Temple. You have returned to Abravanel Hall and this walk's starting point.

POINTS OF INTEREST (START TO FINISH)

Abravanel Hall 123 W. South Temple; for ticket information: ArtTix, arttix.org, 801-355-ARTS (2787); 888-451-ARTS (2787)

City Creek Center shopcitycreekcenter.com, 50 S. Main St., 801-521-2012

Utah Woolen Mills utahwoolenmills.com, 59 W. South Temple, 801-364-1851

Blue Lemon bluelemon.com, 55 W. South Temple, 801-328-2583

Hagermann's Bakehouse Café hagermanns.com, 15 W. South Temple, 801-320-9562

O.C. Tanner octannerstore.com, 15 S. State St., 801-532-3222

Naked Fish Bistro nakedfishbistro.com, 67 W. 100 South

Utah Artist Hands utahands.com, 61 W. 100 South, 801-355-0206

Caffé Molise caffemolise.com, 55 W. 100 South, 801-364-8833

Gallivan Center thegallivancenter.com, 239 S. Main St., 801-535-6110

KUTV connect2utah.com, 299 S. Main St., Ste. 150, 801-839-1234

Capitol Theatre 50 W. 200 South, 801-323-6800; for ticket information: ArtTix, arttix.org, 801-355-ARTS (2787); 888-451-ARTS (2787)

Salt Lake Convention and Visitors Bureau/Visit Salt Lake visitsaltlake.com, 90 S. West Temple, 801-534-4900 or 800-541-4955

Salt Lake Art Center utahmoca.org, 20 S. West Temple, 801-328-4201

route summary

1. Begin at Abravanel Hall, at the southwest corner of West Temple and South Temple, and walk east, crossing West Temple.

2. Continue east along the south side of South Temple to Main St.

3. Cross Main St., continuing east to State St.

4. Turn right at the southeast corner, walking downhill along State St.'s east side to the midblock Social Hall underground tunnel entrance and museum.

5. Using the underground tunnel, head west under State St. via the escalators or stairs to the City Creek Center East food court area.

6. Exit the foot court into City Creek Center's main plaza.

7. Use the escalators, stairways, or elevators to reach the second level above the plaza.

8. On level two, turn left to walk among the shops, crossing Main St. via a sky bridge into City Creek Center West.

9. Continue west on the upper level to the area's circular plaza and descend to ground level.

10. Resume the walk west through the Nordstrom department store and outside to West Temple.

11. On West Temple, turn left to walk south to 100 South. Cross to the intersection's southeast corner.

12. Turn left again to stroll along the south side of 100 South to Main St. and cross to the southeast corner to continue eastward.

13. At Regent St. (50 East), turn right to walk south.

14. At 200 South, use a signaled crosswalk to cross to the Gallivan Center park and performance venue.

15. Veer right at the park's center, between the Utah One and Wells Fargo office towers, walking west toward the Main St. exit.

16. Turn right to walk north on Main St. to 200 South; cross to the intersection's northeast corner, then again to the northwest corner.

17. Continue west for one block, crossing West Temple to the intersection's northwest corner.

18. Turn right to walk one block north beside the Calvin L. Rampton Salt Palace Convention Center, to Abravanel Hall, where this walk began.

CONNECTING THE WALKS

Connect with Walk 1, Temple Square, anywhere between West Temple and State St. on the north side of South Temple along this route.

Connect with Walk 2, Main Street, which includes the north-south axis of City Creek Center and continues to 400 South and back.

Connect with Walk 4, Library Square, the southern downtown area, at the nearby intersection of 300 South and State St.

Connect with Walk 5, West Downtown, at 200 South and West Temple.

Connect with Walk 9, East South Temple, at the Alta Club, on the southeast corner of South Temple and State St.

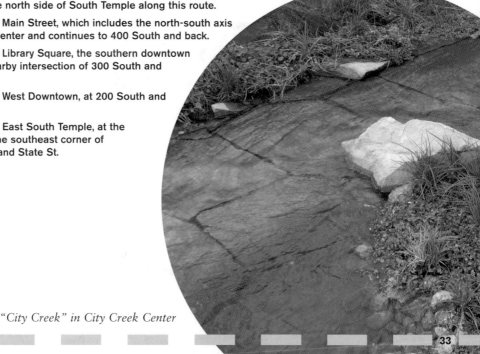

"City Creek" in City Creek Center

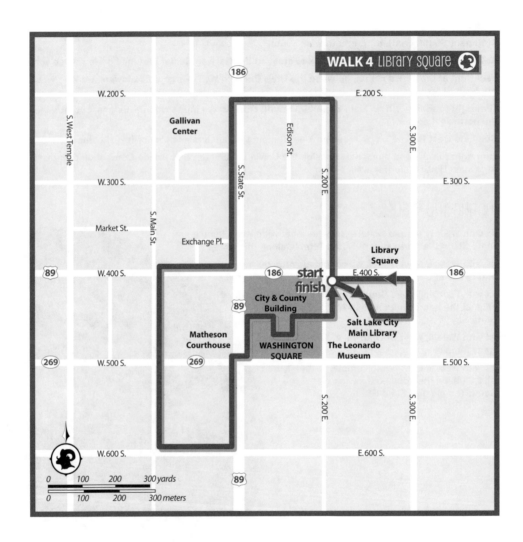

WALK 4 LIBRARY SQUARE

186

W. 200 S.   E. 200 S.

S. West Temple

Gallivan
Center

Edison St.

S. State St.

S. 200 E.

S. 300 E.

W. 300 S.   E. 300 S.

S. Main St.

Market St.

Exchange Pl.

Library
Square

89

W. 400 S.   E. 400 S.   186

186   **start
finish**

89   **City & County
Building**   Salt Lake City
Main Library

**Matheson
Courthouse**   The Leonardo
Museum

269   **WASHINGTON
SQUARE**

269   W. 500 S.   E. 500 S.

S. 200 E.

S. 300 E.

W. 600 S.   E. 600 S.

0   100   200   300 yards

0   100   200   300 meters

89

4 LIBrary Square: BOOK NOOKS aND BOOK 'em

BOUNDARIES: **300 East, 200 South, Main St., and 600 South**
DISTANCE: **2 miles**
DIFFICULTY: **Easy**
PARKING: **Metered street parking; the Main Library's underground parking, accessed at midblock on 400 South eastbound, is free for the first half hour, then $1.50 per half hour.**
PUBLIC TRANSIT: **TRAX light-rail's Library Station is on 400 South, north of the library; TRAX is also on Main St. along a portion of this walk.**

The southern reaches of central downtown Salt Lake City exude civic pride as well as civic order. Here, with 400 South as its axis, you'll find the community's curvaceous new Main Library, its stately City & County Building, the principal district courthouse, and the elegant Grand America Hotel all mixed into an eclectic tapestry of buildings of many ages and businesses of many kinds.

Adjacent blocks Library Square and Washington Square roil with activity year-round, and not simply for their primary roles. Library Square is home to the city's much-praised book heaven, of course, as well as The Leonardo—the "old library," which has been transformed into a multidisciplinary arts, science, and technology museum. Washington Square's centerpiece is the clock-towered, 19th-century city hall, more properly the City & County Building. Intervening 200 East is occasionally shut down to more effectively link the two 10-acre squares, allowing thousands to gather for such celebrations as the multiethnic Living Traditions Festival, the Utah Pride Festival, and the Utah Arts Festival. Adding to the sense of a civic triptych here is the Scott M. Matheson Courthouse, named for the state's 12th governor, which faces the City & County Building from its perch across State St. to the west.

Also nearby are some of Salt Lake City's principal hotel havens, making this downtown section an attractive walking route for travelers yearning to stretch their legs. The gleaming Grand America, a 775-room, AAA Five Diamond hotel, towers to the southwest at 555 S. Main St., east of its elder sibling, the Little America. Both West Temple and 600 South, to the west, are lined with hostelries that include two Hiltons, a Sheraton, a Shilo Inn, and the ageless Peery, more than a hundred years old. The ritzy Hotel Monaco is on Main. TRAX light-rail lines trundle down the centers of both 400 South and Main St. Mid-downtown to the TRAX Library and Courthouse stations is a Free Fare Zone to boot.

With all this potential mobility and numerous hotels, a walk could start most anywhere, but let's make a choice: Library Square and the innovative Main Library itself.

- Begin at the Main Library's principal entrance, 210 E. 400 South, on the southeast corner of the intersection of 200 East and 400 South. Step inside to discover the spacious Urban Room. The glitzy, glass-enclosed atrium seems almost like being in the open air, and the light is definitely natural. The sloping outer wall soars five stories overhead, as glass elevators zip floor to floor like small see-through spaceships. Unlike at your average library, the smell of fresh-roasted coffee and other treats may tease your nose. While library counters and stacks are quite visible beyond the south wall, the atrium itself actually has several shops, offering coffee (of course), sandwiches, books, stationery, and local art. If you have the time, explore the library's collections, head up to and admire the rooftop garden, and walk down the outer Crescent Wall on the structure's east side.

- Library Square itself is worth a leisurely look. The Leonardo, which housed the Main Library from 1964 and for 40 years thereafter, is to the south. Beneath the Crescent Wall are more shops and offices, including a studio for the public radio station KCPW, a community writing center, and Night Flight Comics, which plays a role in the library's effort to encourage children to read. Head toward the square's southeast corner, where walkways pass metallic statuary. One depicts the good old days: two children doing cartwheels, slingshots in their pockets.

- At the corner of 300 East and 500 South, turn left to walk north to 400 South. Much of Library Square, beyond its paved plazas, features both lush flower gardens and xeriscaping, with plants and bushes that require little water. Upon reaching 400 South, turn left again to return west to the library's main entry area, the corner of 200 East and 400 South.

- Turn right to cross 400 South. For reference, there's a Burger King on the intersection's northeast corner. Walk north on 200 East's east side for one block and cross 300 South as well. On the opposite side of 200 East is another of the area's prime

Back Story

In the few years since their grand debut, Salt Lake City's curving crystal Main Library and Library Square have become dynamic public spaces. In fact, in 2006 the facility was named *Library Journal*'s national "Library of the Year"—and Utahns would probably say it deserves the title annually.

The new six-story Main Library was, in fact, designed by the lead architect, internationally renowned Moshe Safdie, and his team to be a strikingly democratic city centerpiece, a focal point for public exchange and inquiry, then–library director Nancy Tessman told LibraryJournal.com in 2006. "The building reflects the idea of an open mind. There are 360-degree views of the city from it. You can look outward in every direction," she said.

The city's citizens approved an $84 million bond for this project and others in 1998, the old Metropolitan Hall of Justice was razed, and ground was broken in 2000. A modernist landmark rose at 210 E. 400 South that opened in 2003, with more than 240,000 square feet of space, more

than a half million books, videos, CDs, and DVDs—and 176,368 square feet of glass, including the sloping, many-paned atrium lens of the Urban Room, skylights, wall windows, doors, and even handrails. A sweeping inclined Crescent Wall rises (or descends!) from the paved central plaza to the library's gardenlike roof, sprinkled with grassy plots, small trees, and flowers.

The library is at once large and cozy. Despite its size, the various levels are rife with sunny desk reading areas, group seating, and computer stations. Unlike many traditional libraries, the complex includes beverage and snack stands and shops, spiral fireplaces, small art and book stores, and, at its east entrance, a comic-book and graphic-novel shop that complements the library's own larger than usual 'zine and graphic-novel collection.

This is not your brick-and-mortar library of the past. Architect Safdie declared the overall goal during the Main Library's grand opening: "My ambition," he said, "was for it to be the best library in the world."

book nooks, this time a shop: Ken Sanders Rare Books, an old industrial building transformed into a treasure chest. Sanders is known for his antiquarian expertise (he's been an expert on public television's *Antiques Roadshow*) and newsworthy offerings. Also here is the cleverly named Tavernacle Social Club, with other interesting shops in a string along 300 South to the east.

● Continue walking north. First United Methodist Church, built in 1905, is on the southeast corner of 200 South and 200 East, reflected in a glass skyscraper looming at its back. (As an optional extension, another block farther north is an even older non-Mormon landmark, St. Mark's Episcopal Cathedral at 231 E. 100 South, built in 1874.)

● At the Methodist meetinghouse, turn right on 200 South to walk west. Dramatically, a colorful pop-art wall mural of Mary, the mother of Jesus, covers the side of one downtown building, high above an eclectic mix of businesses: a gun store, the Cedars of Lebanon Restaurant, Este New York–style pizzeria, and a bank. Across the street is the old Stratford Hotel (now the "Second and Second" building), a cycling shop, a tailor, and a couple of taverns (Johnny's on Second and Bar X).

● At the corner of 200 South and State St., cross State St. and turn left to head south. At 260 S. State St. is the façade of the Brooks Arcade building. Originally built in 1891 by a Jewish businessman and pioneer, the building's interior was razed and its brownstone exterior restored. Today it houses shops and condominiums and serves as the AlphaGraphics photocopy chain's world headquarters.

● Continue south on State St., crossing Exchange Place (355 South). In the block's center, to the west, is Salt Lake City's old Wall Street–like stock exchange district (described as part of Walk 2, Main Street). Continue south to 400 South. On the corner is the century-old former Hotel Plandome, originally a labor hall.

● Cross 400 South to its south side. Before you is the modern and very busy Matheson Courthouse, which includes district and juvenile courtrooms, the Utah Supreme Court, and state administrative law offices.

● Turn right to proceed west on 400 South to Main St. On the corner, at 405 S. Main St., towers the sleek steel-and-glass First Security Bank Building, now headquarters for Utah's Ken Garff auto dealership empire. Though once considered by some critics to be the modernist "ugly duckling" of Salt Lake skycrapers, the 12-story 1950s tower is today generally deemed "retro cool." The building is significant: As a historical marker notes, it was the city's first new high-rise after a two-decade-plus dry spell in the wake of the Great Depression. In midintersection at 400 South and Main St. you'll note that the TRAX light-rail lines diverge, with one route heading south to bisect the Salt Lake Valley and another heading east toward the University of Utah.

● Turn left on Main St. and walk south. The TRAX Courthouse Station is at midblock. Carefully cross 500 South, a traffic-heavy, one-way access to I-15 and I-80 to the west. At 555 S. Main St. rises the Grand America, a five-star hotel completed prior to the 2002 Winter Olympic Games, hosted by Salt Lake City. At 24 stories tall, it boasts 775 rooms and 1.2 million square feet of space. Consider stepping inside. Designed to be a European-style boutique hotel, albeit on a massive American scale, it boasts Italian-made chandeliers, French cherry-wood furniture, English wool carpets, and bathrooms of Italian marble. Across Main St. is the block-filling Little America Hotel, an older sister property of hotel and Sinclair Oil owner Earl Holding, with another 850 rooms.

● At 600 South, turn left to walk east, still navigating around the Grand America's huge footprint. Across the street to the south is the Studio 600 dance club. Turn left again at State St., proceeding one block north. Cross 500 South toward the Matheson Courthouse; then turn right at the same intersection to cross State St. at 500 South to the southwest tip of Washington Square.

● Walk north to the middle of the block, marked by a pole and monument honoring the U.S. flag and U.S. Constitution, with 1930s-era statues of a girl and a boy. Turn right and step toward the historic Salt Lake City & County Building, the square's only structure. Built from 1892 to 1894, this is Salt Lake's city hall, though it originally housed both city and county administrations—and served as Utah's first state capitol, from 1896 to 1915. The Kyune sandstone building reflects the Romanesque Revival architectural tradition. But the City & County Building has an almost medieval effect. Gargoyles hover overhead. Creatures lurk, from mythological dragons to wary lizards. And there are faces galore: actual portraits and dozens of others, including masklike visages of pioneers and Indians. In the 1980s the structure underwent a $30 million restoration, a process that added 443 base isolators to help absorb the shock of an earthquake registering up to 7.0 on the Richter scale. The grounds are shaded, with gardens and fountains. The building is open during business hours, so enter the west doors and cut through the tiled center hall. Tours are offered Tuesdays at noon, June through August, by the Utah Heritage Foundation. On the building's east side is a separate entrance into the Washington Square Café, a little countertop eatery reminiscent of another time.

● Once outside, walk east and cross 200 East at midblock, where there is a pedestrian signal. The Leonardo is on the corner south of Salt Lake City's new Main Library. The former library reopened in 2011 as a culture, arts, and science center. Visit its exhibits, if you wish. You have returned to Library Square, where this walk began.

POINTS OF INTEREST (START TO FINISH)

Main Library www.slcpl.lib.ut.us, 210 E. 400 South, 801-524-8200

The Leonardo theleonardo.org, 300 S. 500 East, 801-531-9800

Night Flight Comics night-flight.com, 210 E. 400 South, 801-532-1188

Ken Sanders Rare Books kensandersbooks.com, 268 S. 200 East, 801-521-3819

Tavernacle Social Club tavernaclenightclub.com, 201 E. 300 South, 801-833-0570

First United Methodist Church firstmethodistslc.org, 203 E. 200 South, 801-328-8726

St. Mark's Episcopal Cathedral stmarkscathedral-ut.org, 231 E. 100 South, 801-322-3400

Cedars of Lebanon Restaurant cedarsoflebanonrestaurant.com, 150 E. 200 South, 801-364-4096

Este Pizzeria estepizzaco.com, 156 E. 200 South, 801-363-2366

Johnny's on Second johnnysonsecond.com, 165 E. 200 South, 801-746-3334

Bar X 155 E. 200 South, 801-532-9114

Grand America Hotel grandamerica.com, 555 S. Main St., 800-304-8696

Little America Hotel littleamerica.com, 500 S. Main St., 800-281-7899

Studio 600 Dance Club mystudio600.com, 26 E. 600 South, 801-355-9860

Salt Lake City & County Building slcclassic.com/government, 451 S. State St., 801-535-6333

Washington Square Café 451 S. State St., 801-535-6102

route summary

1. Start at Salt Lake City's Main Library, on the northwest corner of Library Square, 200 East and 400 South. Visit the library and make your way to the block's southeast corner, 300 East and 500 South. (If the library is not open, circle the building to the east and south.)

2. Walk north on 300 East to 400 South, turn left to walk west, and return to 200 East and 400 South.

3. Walk north for two blocks, crossing 400 South and 300 South to 200 South.

4. Turn left at 200 South, cross 200 East, and proceed one block to State St.

5. At the corner of 200 South and State St., cross State St. and turn left to head south.

6. At 400 South, turn right and proceed west for one block to Main St.

7. Turn left to cross 400 South (a complicated intersection with diverging TRAX light-rail lines) and continue south for two blocks to 600 South.

8. Turn left to walk east on 600 South to State St., then turn left again to walk north, crossing 500 South to the Matheson Courthouse.

9. Turn right and cross State St. to the southwest corner of Washington Square.

10. Turn left, walk north a half block, then turn right toward the City & County Building. Meander Washington Square, examining the historic building's carvings, but return to the building's west entrance.

11. If it's open, shortcut through the City & County Building; otherwise circle the building to its east side, where there is a midblock pedestrian crossing.

12. Cross 200 East to Library Square, home of The Leonardo museum and the Main Library, where this walk began.

Connecting the Walks

Connect with Walk 2, Main Street, at 400 South.

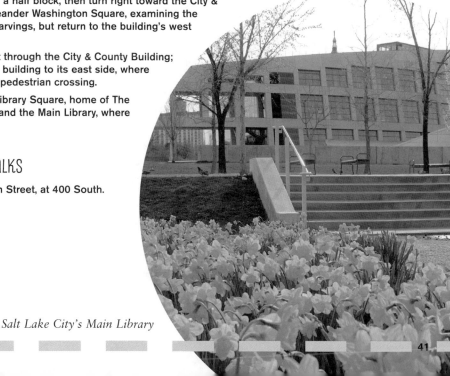

Salt Lake City's Main Library

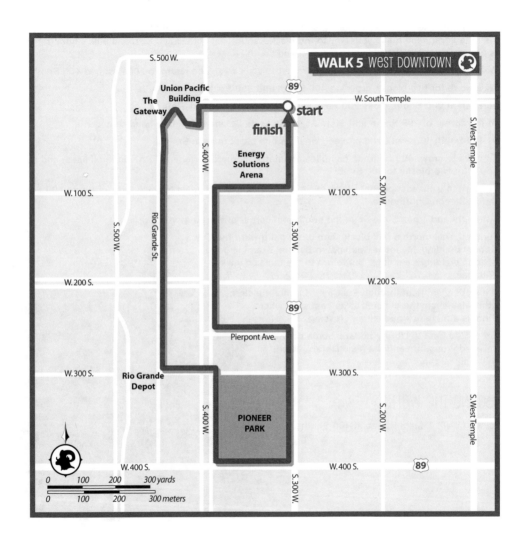

WALK 5 WEST DOWNTOWN

S. 500 W.

Union Pacific
Building

The
Gateway

start

finish

W. South Temple

S. West Temple

Energy
Solutions
Arena

S. 400 W.

W. 100 S.

S. 500 W.

Rio Grande St.

S. 300 W.

W. 100 S.

S. 200 W.

W. 200 S.

W. 200 S.

S. 300 W.

Pierpont Ave.

W. 300 S.

Rio Grande
Depot

S. 400 W.

W. 300 S.

S. 200 W.

S. West Temple

PIONEER
PARK

W. 400 S.

W. 400 S.

S. 300 W.

0   100   200   300 yards

0   100   200   300 meters

5 WEST DOWNTOWN: THE GATEWAY AND ALL THAT JAZZ

BOUNDARIES: **South Temple, Rio Grande St., 400 South, and 300 West**
DISTANCE: **3 miles**
DIFFICULTY: **Easy**
PARKING: **The Gateway mall has a large underground parking terrace, with validation available at most stores and restaurants; entrances are on 400 West and on 200 South; an outdoor lot is on the mall's north side, and metered street parking is available.**
PUBLIC TRANSIT: **TRAX light-rail parallels The Gateway's east and south sides via the Arena, Planetarium, and Old Greek Town stations.**

For much of the 21st century's first decade, The Gateway proved to be Salt Lake City's alternate downtown. The city's traditional commercial heart, south of Temple Square, was a massive construction zone as the new City Creek Center was being born. The Gateway, however, was the community's first modern open-air shopping mall, having opened in 2001 on downtown's western fringe. It has since become a premier gathering place, with a tony central artery, office buildings, and more than 100 stores and restaurants. It plays host to popular annual events, such as the St. Patrick's Day Parade, the holiday lighting, and the final leg of the Salt Lake City Marathon.

The Gateway debuted just prior to the 2002 Winter Olympic Games, which were hosted by the city. A circular cobblestone area draws shoppers and their children (in summer, often in swimsuits) to a centerpiece of that heady time, Olympic Legacy Plaza and its fountain. It is thrilling still to be there when upward-shooting columns of water begin dancing to a recording of a Mormon Tabernacle Choir and Utah Symphony performance of composer John Williams' Olympic theme. The choir forcefully voices the Olympic motto: *"Citius! Altius! Fortius!"*—Latin for faster, higher, and stronger.

The broader Gateway District has been in the midst of gentrification. The area remains a center for services to the homeless. Be cautiously aware that shelters are nearby. Historic Pioneer Park is a magnet for transients in daytime—yet is also popular with all when it hosts the Farmers Market and occasional concert. Another big attraction, the 20,000-seat Energy

Solutions Arena, is home of the NBA's Utah Jazz (twice a title contender in the late 1990s), as well as many major concerts and other events. The Gateway also includes Clark Planetarium and the Discover Gateway Children's Museum.

History abounds. This is Salt Lake City's onetime Greek town. The Greek Orthodox church is here, as is the community's historic railroad hub. The century-old Union Pacific and Rio Grande depots still proudly stand and serve the community, albeit for other purposes, and bookend the district on the north and south. That mobile tradition continues, with the area's transportation hub, Salt Lake Central Station, a block away, on 600 West and 200 South. TRAX light-rail, FrontRunner commuter rail, and bus routes all converge at this modern terminal.

● Begin this walk at the northwest corner of South Temple and 300 West, across the street from the Energy Solutions Arena. This block is principally occupied by the Triad Center, a business, media, and education complex. TRAX light-rail's Arena Station is in the center of South Temple, complete with a clock-monument commemorating the 2002 Winter Olympic Games.

● Stroll west on South Temple, toward 400 West, on the street's north side. At midblock, amid a manicured landscape, sits the antique Devereaux House, the oldest structure on this side of town and Salt Lake City's earliest mansion. Portions date to 1855, when it was built by pioneer William Staines in a cottage style, complete with English gardens reminiscent of his homeland. The residence was greatly expanded and remodeled in the 1870s by William Jennings. A merchant, Jennings became Utah's first millionaire, and he was elected mayor in 1882. Elegant and spacious for a frontier community, Devereaux House hosted elaborate dinners during its 19th-century heyday. Presidents Ulysses S. Grant and Rutherford B. Hayes, as well as General William Tecumseh Sherman, were among the guests. After the Transcontinental Railroad came to Utah, this became more of a business and industrial area, and Devereaux House went into decline. It was restored in the 1970s to again serve as a dining and reception center.

● At 400 West, cross to the west side of the street. This is the Gateway retail area. Salt Lake City's Union Pacific train station, with an iconic red, white, and blue neon shield, dominates the head of South Temple. The facility is no longer a railroad terminal. A concert venue, The Depot, is on its northern end. The great hall is used for weddings, corporate events, and concerts and is a grand entrance to The Gateway; use it as such, unless some other event has closed the terminal to the public. Built in 1909 at a cost of $450,000, the cavernous depot and its long benches may no longer throng with rail passengers, but evocative murals remain, depicting scenes of the pioneers and the meeting of the transcontinental rails at Promontory Summit, Utah, in 1869.

● If the depot is closed, enter The Gateway south of the Union Pacific building. Note Fleming's Prime Steakhouse & Wine Bar at 20 S. 400 West. Turn left at the Gateway sign about midblock, where there is a gap between buildings. The walkway curves as you proceed west, passing various businesses, including a souvenir shop. Whether you entered The Gateway via the terminal or the sidewalk, you are now above the Olympic Legacy Plaza. Stone stairways lead down to the gathering place and fountain. A gigantic version of the 2002 Games' symbol is rendered in tiles upon which the fountain waters dance and spray. Brick memorials and placards honor Games contributors, and a dynamic *Go for the Gold* skiing statue is to the northwest.

● Walk to the nearby street, Rio Grande, which bisects The Gateway. Go left (south) to meander past assorted businesses—stores and boutiques both well known and specialized, selling apparel, sporting goods, eyewear, shoes, and home furnishings. This is a substantial all-seasons mall, with retail establishments both at street level and arrayed along a second-story promenade, accessible via stairways, elevators, and an escalator. Discovery Gateway, a children's museum, is on the northeast corner of Rio Grande and 100 South. Just to the east, at 100 South and 400 West, is the Clark Planetarium and an IMAX 3-D theater. On the second level toward The Gateway's south

Union Pacific depot

Back Story

Despite a checkered history, Salt Lake City's Pioneer Park has an honored place in Utah history. Here, in 1847, the Mormon pioneers built their first settlement in the Salt Lake Valley—a 10-acre walled fort. At the end of a 1,000-mile migration from the area of what is today Council Bluffs, Iowa, and Omaha, Nebraska, more than 2,000 pioneers from multiple wagon trains took shelter in rough huts to spend the winter of 1847–1848. This has been called, as a bronze Daughter of Utah Pioneers marker notes, "the Plymouth Rock of the West," the first Anglo-Saxon settlement in the Great Basin and beyond.

In the area of today's Pioneer Park the settlers held their first school classes (for six students), built a bowery for church services and public meetings, and raised the American flag—though this was still technically Mexican territory, and the United States and Mexico were at war to the south. In 1848, Mexico ceded, for peace and payment of $15 million and assumption of $3.25 in debt, much of what is today the American West—basically Utah, California, Nevada, and Arizona and parts of Wyoming, New Mexico, and Colorado—to the United States in the Treaty of Guadalupe Hidalgo.

Settlers soon began moving away, setting up more permanent homes, gardens, and farm fields in what they at first called Great Salt Lake City, in what they hoped would be the State of Deseret.

The fort's structures were dismantled in the early 1850s, after leaders realized they were being used by persons with loose morals—a bad reputation that would come back to haunt the site by the end of the 20th century, when the block became a haven for transients and drug dealers.

The Old Fort settlement became Pioneer Park on Pioneer Day, July 24, 1898. Playgrounds, swimming pools, and picnic grounds soon followed. Although still frequented by some homeless and transients, police are vigilant in the area, and recent renovation has improved the setting, bringing new businesses to occupy nearby buildings. As part of the park's resurgence, it hosts a substantial seasonal Farmers Market. The market sets up booths and tents on Saturdays from June to October and on Tuesdays from August to October.

The city also presents a summer concerts, free outdoor movie screenings, and other events.

end, beyond 100 South, are the Megaplex 12 theaters (on the east) and an indoor food court (on the west), assembling many of the usual suspects, from Taco Time to McDonald's. The Gateway also has towers with offices and condominiums.

● At 200 South and Rio Grande, The Gateway's southern thoroughfare, there is no signalized crossing. There are intersection signals to the west (500 West) and the east (400 West). Caution is advised crossing here, since besides motorized traffic, eastbound and westbound TRAX light-rail trains also regularly pass by. Across the way, on the south side of the street, is the crossroads for Utah's homeless population. Some walkers may feel uncomfortable for half a block here. Remember: There is safety in numbers. The Road Home Shelter is on the west side of Rio Grande, and the Catholic St. Vincent de Paul dining hall is on the east side. Both charities cater to those in need.

● Continue south on Rio Grande. A block away, facing east toward 300 South, is Salt Lake City's historic Rio Grande Depot, home of the Denver & Rio Grande Western Railroad for most of the 20th century. The first trains departed from the then-new terminal in August 1910. The Beaux Arts–Renaissance Revival exterior is grand, but if the depot is open when you drop by, step inside. Today the depot houses the Utah Historical Society, the State Archives, and the visual and public art programs of the Utah Division of Arts and Museums. On the depot's north side is the Rio Grande Café, a popular Tex-Mex restaurant with décor that blends both the railroad past and the arty present. Bustling with travelers and well-wishers 50 years ago, today the main Rio Grande hall is a quiet museum space. Art is often on display, including paintings and photographs of the depot's and Salt Lake City's past. A brick plaza is outside on the depot's west side, where locomotives once chugged, puffed, and hulked, the heroic essence of mechanized power.

● After admiring the Rio Grande Depot, continue from the depot's front entrance, walking east on the north side of 300 South. The old Park (Rio Grande) Hotel along this block once provided housing and services for blue-collar workers, most of them immigrants employed in transportation or related work in the area. Other small hotels from the railroad era are sprinkled along nearby streets. A modern multistory successor, the Homewood Suites, has risen across the street to maintain the tradition.

- Walk to 400 West and cross to the east. Then turn right and cross 300 South to stroll south along the western border of the block-filling, 10-acre Pioneer Park on 400 West to 400 South. Continue on a sidewalk path that will just about circumnavigate the block, turning left at 300 West to walk north along the park's eastern boundary. (For more information on Pioneer Park, see this chapter's Back Story.) Continue north to 300 South.

- Cross 300 South. On the intersection's northwest corner is the 1925 brown-brick Firestone Tire & Rubber Company building, a thriving enterprise in the early years of the automotive age. The building and adjoining structures now house food emporiums with an Italian flavor: the much-praised Cucina Toscana restaurant (two proud bronze pigs and a piglet pose outside), Carlucci's Bakery, and Tony Caputo's Market & Deli. "Tire Town" also includes lofts and condominiums. Across 300 West, reflecting a traditional Byzantine style in brick, is the Holy Trinity Greek Orthodox Church. A Utah historic site, this "Greek Town" church began serving the immigrant district in 1924, especially miners, railroad and smelter workers, and their families, who were lured to Utah by jobs during an era of rapid industrialization.

- Walk north along 300 West, and at midblock turn left on Pierpont Ave. (250 South). A slightly faded mural painted on an east-facing wall pays pastel tribute to laborers and artisans: muscular construction workers as well as a woman pottery maker. To the north is the light-brown Crane Building, a five-story office structure built in 1911 for the international plumbing and heating giant. Stroll west on quirky Pierpont, redeveloped by Artspace as a midcity home to architects, artists, and art galleries. Today the former Free Farmers' Market Building, originally constructed in 1910 to house wholesale produce companies, encompasses 30 studios, 23 residences, and a variety of offices and stores. You may note to the north another industrial building from the past, renovated for modern uses. Toward the roof, in white-on-black block letters, aging paint advertises the California Tire and Rubber Company.

- At 400 West, note across the street the colorful urban mural *SLC Pepper,* artist Jann Haworth's pop-art tribute to The Beatles' *Sgt. Pepper's Lonely Hearts Club Band* album cover—itself a pop-art classic in which she had a designing hand.

- Turn right and walk north. At the southeast corner of 200 South and 400 West is the historic Henderson block, Salt Lake's first produce warehouse area, built in 1909. Vintage "Cornwall Warehouse" lettering graces the top of the building.

- Cross 200 South at the signal and continue walking north. We've returned to The Gateway's precincts, and across 400 West are the mall's movie theaters and its restaurant row, with several options, from family dining (Applebee's, California Pizza Kitchen) to white linen (Biaggi's Ristorante Italiano), as well as coffee shops and grills. Enterprises along the street's west side include the Clark Planetarium, *The Salt Lake Tribune,* and Dick's Sporting Goods.

- Cross 100 South and 400 West to the intersection's northeast corner and turn right, walking east for one block along the south side of the capacious Energy Solutions Arena. Turn left at the corner of 100 South and 300 West into a plaza and garden. The highlights are separate statues of two basketball greats, the effective "pick and roll" duo of retired NBA superstars Karl Malone and John Stockton. The Utah Jazz power forward and point guard, respectively—both now in the NBA Hall of Fame—are the subjects of *Special Delivery* and *Threading the Needle,* by sculptor Brian Challis.

- Continue north along 300 West, the 1991 arena's primary face, to South Temple. You've returned to the TRAX line's Arena Station and the intersection where this walk began.

POINTS OF INTEREST (START TO FINISH)

Energy Solutions Arena energysolutionsarena.com, 301 W. South Temple, 801-325-2000

Devereaux House templesquarehospitality.com/mansion/weddings, 340 W. South Temple, 800-881-5762

The Gateway shopthegateway.com, 18 N. Rio Grande St., 801-456-2000

The Depot depotslc.com, 13 N. 400 West, 801-456-2800

Fleming's Prime Steakhouse & Wine Bar flemingssteakhouse.com, 20 S. 400 West, #2020, 801-355-3704

Discover Gateway Children's Museum discoverygateway.org, 444 W. 100 South, 801-456-5437

Clark Planetarium clarkplanetarium.org, 110 S. 400 West, 801-456-7827

Rio Grande Depot history.utah.gov/about_us/depot.html, 300 S. Rio Grande St., 801-533-3500

Rio Grande Café 270 S. Rio Grande St., 801-364-3302

Pioneer Park slcclassic.com/publicservices/parks/parkspages/Pioneer.htm, 300 S. 300 West

Cucina Toscana cucina-toscana.com, 308 W. 300 South, 801-328-3463

Carlucci's Bakery carluccisbakery.com, 314 W. Broadway, #1, 801-366-4484

Tony Caputo's Market & Deli caputosdeli.com, 314 W. 300 South, 801-531-8669

Holy Trinity Greek Orthodox Church gocslc.org, 279 S. 300 West, 801-328-9681

Applebee's applebees.com, 159 S. Rio Grande St., #1018, 801-456-5000

California Pizza Kitchen cpk.com, 156 S. 400 West, 801-456-0075

Biaggi's Ristorante Italiano biaggis.com, 194 S. 400 West, 801-596-7222

Utah Transit Authority's Salt Lake Central Station rideuta.com, (TRAX, FrontRunner rail, buses), 600 W. 250 South, 801-743-3882

route summary

1. Start at the northwest corner of South Temple and 300 West, walking west on South Temple.

2. Cross at 400 West and either walk through the Union Pacific building (if open) or turn left to midblock and then right (west) into the Gateway shopping complex.

3. Visit Olympic Legacy Plaza and fountain; then turn left to walk south on Rio Grande St. or on the second-level promenade, meandering among the mall's shops.

4. Walk south on Rio Grande, crossing 100 South and then 200 South (carefully, as there is no signal light here, though there are signals at 400 West and 500 West).

5. Continue walking south on Rio Grande St. to the Rio Grande Depot. Visit the terminal, or turn left to proceed east on the north side of 300 South.

6. Walk to 400 West, cross the street to the east, then turn right to walk south on 400 West along the western border of Pioneer Park.

7. Continue to 400 South, turn left at the corner to walk east to 300 West, and then turn left again to walk north up 300 West.

8. Cross 300 South, continuing north to midblock Pierpont Ave. at 250 South, and turn left to walk west.

9. At 400 West, turn right to walk north, crossing intersections at 200 South and 100 South.

10. At 100 South turn right, walking one block east beside Energy Solutions Arena to 300 West.

11. Turn left at 300 West and return to the starting point on South Temple.

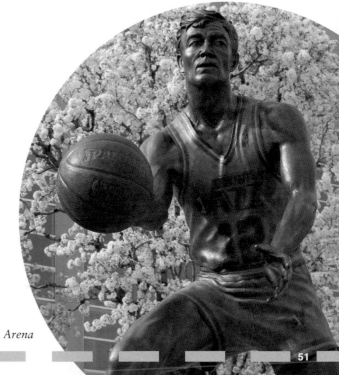

John Stockton statue at Energy Solutions Arena

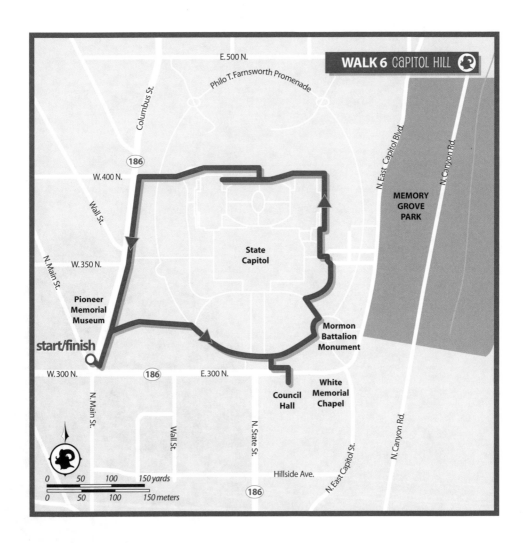

E. 500 N.

Philo T. Farnsworth Promenade

Columbus St.

186

W. 400 N.

Wall St.

N. Main St.

W. 350 N.

State Capitol

Pioneer Memorial Museum

start/finish

W. 300 N.

186

E. 300 N.

N. Main St.

Wall St.

N. State St.

Mormon Battalion Monument

Council Hall

White Memorial Chapel

N. East Capitol St.

Hillside Ave.

N. Canyon Rd.

186

N. East Capitol Blvd.

N. Canyon Rd.

MEMORY GROVE PARK

| 0 | 50 | 100 | 150 yards |
| 0 | 50 | 100 | 150 meters |

6 CAPITOL HILL: a CAPITAL CAPITOL EXPERIENCE

BOUNDARIES: **300 North St., North Main St./Columbus St., East Capitol Blvd., and 500 North St.**
DISTANCE: **1.5 miles**
DIFFICULTY: **Moderate**
PARKING: **Free at the Council Hall lot for visitors, at the State Capitol lot, or along East Capitol Blvd. (Parking is unusually sparse during sessions of the Utah legislative session, which begins the fourth Monday in January and lasts through mid-March.)**
PUBLIC TRANSIT: **Within Salt Lake City's Free Fare Zone, UTA bus #500 drops by the Utah State Capitol on weekdays dozens of times each day. The route (which can change due to construction, etc.) is accessible at three points around the Capitol grounds, connecting passengers to the city's downtown, along State St., North Temple, and Main St. Pick up a free route map.**

Utah's elegant State Capitol is grandly perched on aptly named Capitol Hill, just north of downtown Salt Lake City. It is visible from every direction, "its magisterial air emphasized by its elevation 300 feet above the valley floor," notes the 1982 revision of the Depression-era *Utah: A Guide to the State.* To appreciate the building's classic, colonnaded design, nothing is better than a stroll of the grounds, a stroll inside, and visits to historic buildings on its perimeter. What stands out for many visitors (and filmmakers) is that of all the nation's statehouses, Utah's may most closely resemble the U.S. Capitol in Washington, D.C. That evocation was planned: Utah, settled long before most other Western states, fought fiercely for statehood for nearly a half century, and when that goal was finally achieved in 1896, Mormon, non-Mormon, and other factions wanted a building, as Kirk Huffaker observes in his book *Salt Lake City Then and Now,* that reflected their shared desire to be unequivocally deemed part of the United States. Built of Utah granite, like so many of Salt Lake City's major edifices, and completed in 1916 after four years of construction, the 320,000-square-foot building also underwent a four-year seismic upgrade from 2004 to 2008. The result is an expanded complex, based on the early 20th-century plan, with new (yes, granite-faced) House and Senate office buildings and a renovated Capitol that seems sparkling and new. Add in lofty views of the Salt Lake Valley, a reconstructed city hall across the way, a free pioneer museum next door, and a bevy of monuments and you have the ingredients for a most invigorating and enlightening walk.

● Begin at the northwest corner of North Main St. and 300 North, southwest of the State Capitol building. Here, at the top of Salt Lake City's Main St., stands the stately Pioneer Memorial Museum. A statue of pioneer poet and suffragist Eliza R. Snow stands in the midst of a rose garden at the building's front. Inside, exhibited in a close but remarkably orderly fashion, are thousands upon thousands of pioneer artifacts and keepsakes. "It's the best-kept secret in the state of Utah," according to guide Caroleen May, a member of the Daughters of Utah Pioneers, who maintain the museum. Admission is free, and "people are amazed at what we have here," May says. Although no photography is allowed inside, visitors glimpse entire pioneer-era furnished rooms, pins and buttons, china and dishes, quilts, books, musical instruments, maps, tools, dolls, coins, jewelry, clothing—the sheer variety is staggering. Highlights include artifacts belonging to early Mormon Church leaders Joseph Smith and Brigham Young, a gleaming 1902 fire engine, a full-size covered wagon from the late 1850s, pioneer guns and swords, the original eagle from Brigham Young's Eagle Gate, and even Transcontinental Railroad memorabilia. Other artifacts were gathered overseas during the 19th century—from Hawaii, the South Pacific, and China, for instance. Restrooms are available.

● Walk southeast from the Pioneer Museum and cross Main St. at the crosswalk to the State Capitol grounds. Several small monuments and markers grace the grounds here—a "Lest We Forget" memorial to pioneers who died en route to Utah; a monument honoring the U.S. Constitution; another summarizing the history of Ensign Peak, which rises behind the capitol; and another remembering duties fulfilled by Utahns during the relatively distant Civil War, such as protecting the then-new transcontinental telegraph lines.

● Return to and follow the sidewalk along 300 North, past a new concrete wall at the top of State St., its bronze letters declaring "State of Utah," to a crosswalk. Cross the street south to the old Salt Lake City Hall, a cupola-topped red-sandstone civic building originally built downtown from 1864 to 1865. In 1961, as a historical placard notes, the structure was moved "stone by stone, and restored to its original likeness." It now houses the Utah Travel Council, giving the building its current name: Council Hall. Inside are meeting rooms and an everything-Utah-oriented gift shop, offering free tourist information and brochures, as well as maps, postcards, and books.

• Next door to the east is the White Memorial Chapel. This was originally the 1883 Gothic Revival 18th Ward LDS Church meetinghouse, which stood several blocks away. Demolished in 1873, as a historical marker notes, many key parts were salvaged—the steeple, cornerstone, window frames, doors, pulpit, benches, and stained glass—and are featured in this reconstruction, often used for weddings and other special occasions.

• Return to the crosswalk and walk back onto the formal State Capitol grounds. Prominently poised about 50 yards away is a towering and intricate monument celebrating the Mormon Battalion. Its statuary, carvings, and nameplates remember a corps of 500 volunteers recruited during the Mormon trek west to serve in the Mexican-American War of 1846–1848. Among its many accomplishments was one of the longest marches in world military history, 2,000 miles south to New Mexico and then to San Diego and Los Angeles, building a road and digging wells along the way, as the placards observe. Former battalion members were among the first to discover gold in California on January 24, 1848.

• Both sidewalks and a curving garden path lead to the capitol's east entrance. Just outside stands a heroic statue of Massassoit, the Indian leader who was a friend of the pilgrims in Massachusetts. The original statue is, of course, on the East Coast. But as placards note, it was sculpted by Utah artist Cyrus E. Dallin, who presented the plaster cast to the state of Utah in 1922. In 1959 it was cast in bronze and long stood guard at the front of the capitol, until the renovations of 2004, when it was placed here.

• On either side of the capitol's east entry are two majestic Italian-marble lions, named for the virtues "Integrity" and "Fortitude" and carved by artist Nick Fairplay during the renovation to replace their deteriorated concrete predecessors. (Another pair, "Honor" and "Patience," guard the west entrance.) If you have time, certainly step inside the capitol. (If not, walk to the rear of the building and its central courtyard.) This is the statehouse's lower level. Free guided tours are generally available in the daytime. But on your own you can examine historical displays, including the portrait-lined Hall of Governors, and drop by the gift shop. Take the stairs to the main level and admire the rotunda and the evocative cyclorama and pendentive murals below the sky-painted dome. The murals depict such events as the 1776 trek by the Spanish friars Dominguez and Escalante through Utah; American explorer John C. Fremont at the Great Salt Lake; and early trappers and traders, such as Peter Skene Ogden, in northern Utah. Consider stepping out the capitol's huge metal south doors, which presents a majestic view of Salt Lake City on the capitol's front steps, flanked by the building's elegant Corinthian columns. Also inside, on the upper level, are two more early 20th-century murals depicting pioneer-era Salt Lake Valley and the chambers of Utah's House, Senate, and Supreme Court.

● Once you've finished ogling the capitol's traditional yet elegant interior, exit to the west (and the second set of marble lions) or to the north, heading to the grounds' central plaza, which features a reflecting pool and yet more statuary. One is a monument to Brigadier General Thomas L. Kane, a friend and champion of the Mormon pioneers. Another remembers Daniel Cowan Jackling, an innovative metallurgist who developed processes used in modern mass-production copper mining—and organized the Utah Copper Co. and the huge open-pit Bingham Canyon Mine—while a third hails Martha Hughes Cannon, a Utah doctor and medical pioneer, a suffragist, and the first woman elected to a state senate in United States history.

● Stroll to the capitol's western side and slope, where moving memorials honor and name Utah's fallen law enforcement personnel ("Greater love hath no man than this, that a man lay down his life for his friends") and those who served and who died in the Vietnam War of the 1960s and '70s ("They kept the faith. They made the ultimate sacrifice").

● From these thought-provoking memorials, it is a simple stroll south and west, via sidewalk or groomed lawn, to where this walk began: Pioneer Memorial Museum. We've offered a rather roundabout route, rife with possible stops and detours. A walk on the sidewalks on the outer edges of the capitol grounds, beside the roads, would cover about a mile; the grounds encompass a square mile.

POINTS OF INTEREST (START TO FINISH)

Pioneer Memorial Museum dupinternational.org, 300 N. Main St., 801-532-6479, ext. 206

Utah State Capitol utahstatecapitol.utah.gov, 350 N. State St., 801-538-3074

Utah Travel Council travel.utah.gov, 300 N. State St., 801-538-1900

White Memorial Chapel utahstatecapitol.utah.gov, 150 E. 300 North, 801-410-0011

route summary

1. Start at the northwest corner of North Main St. and 300 North (Pioneer Memorial Museum).

2. Walk southeast from the Pioneer Memorial Museum and cross Main St. at the crosswalk to the State Capitol grounds.

3. Explore the historical monuments in the area.

4. Return to the sidewalk along 300 North and walk about 150 yards east to a crosswalk, just beyond the North State St. junction.

5. Cross the street to the south to two historic buildings, Council Hall and White Memorial Chapel.

6. Return to the capitol grounds and pause at the large Mormon Battalion monument in the southeast corner.

7. Walk north toward the capitol's east entrance, entering if it is open, for a look. If not, loop to the plaza at the rear of the building to find three statues and a reflecting pool.

8. Return southwest to the capitol's west side, which features monuments remembering Vietnam veterans and fallen lawmen. Or, if inside the Capitol, exit the front doors for a view; return and exit the west or north doors for the additional memorials.

9. Walk southwest and cross North Main St. to return to this walk's starting point at the Pioneer Memorial Museum.

connecting the walks

Walk down Main St. or State St. to North Temple and connect with Walk 1, Temple Square.

Hillside stairs southeast of the capitol grounds connect with Walk 7, Memory Grove/ City Creek Canyon.

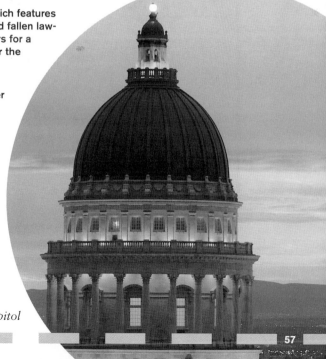

Utah State Capitol

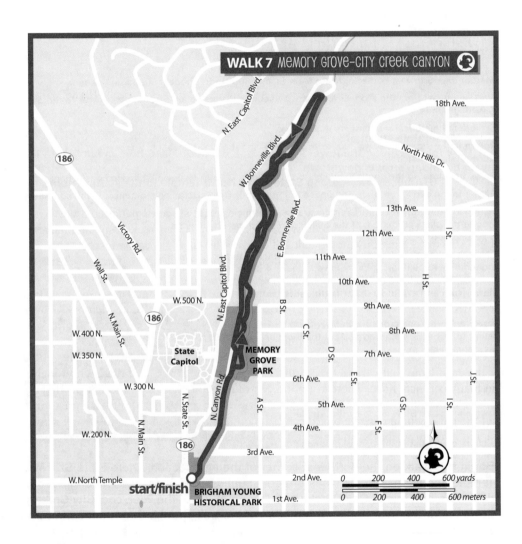

WALK 7 MEMORY GROVE-CITY CREEK CANYON

18th Ave.

N. East Capitol Blvd.

North Hills Dr.

186

W. Bonneville Blvd.

E. Bonneville Blvd.

13th Ave.

12th Ave.

1 St.

11th Ave.

Victory Rd.

10th Ave.

H St.

Wall St.

9th Ave.

W. 500 N.

186

N. East Capitol Blvd.

8th Ave.

N. Main St.

W. 400 N.

B St.

7th Ave.

W. 350 N.

State
Capitol

MEMORY
GROVE
PARK

C St.

D St.

6th Ave.

G St.

1 St.

W. 300 N.

N. Canyon Rd.

E St.

5th Ave.

J St.

A St.

4th Ave.

F St.

N. State St.

N. Main St.

W. 200 N.

186

3rd Ave.

0   200   400   600 yards

2nd Ave.

0   200   400   600 meters

W. North Temple

start/finish BRIGHAM YOUNG
HISTORICAL PARK

1st Ave.

7 MEMORY GROVE/CITY CREEK CANYON: NATURE AT DOWNTOWN'S EDGE

BOUNDARIES: **North Temple–2nd Ave., Canyon Rd., West and East Bonneville Blvds., and East Capitol Blvd.**
DISTANCE: **3.5 miles**
DIFFICULTY: **Moderately strenuous**
PARKING: **Park for free along the lower sections of Canyon Rd.; two-hour metered parking is available along streets downtown.**
PUBLIC TRANSIT: **UTA buses travel along State St. or North Temple to the starting point.**

Skyscrapers, traffic, noise, and congestion—then a peaceful, secluded park and a near-wilderness. Such is the contrast presented by Memory Grove and lower City Creek Canyon, a narrow oasis only blocks from teeming downtown Salt Lake City. This is an all-season favorite of walkers, dogs, joggers, and bicyclists, as traffic is banned from most of the route. For early settlers City Creek was an invaluable, safeguarded source of water for the infant city, providing water for people, animals, and the first farm fields. It remains a prime drinking-water resource. The community's first mills were here. Near the canyon mouth today is gardenlike Memory Grove, set aside as a park in 1902 and dedicated in 1924 as a memorial to soldiers lost in World War I. This was originally Memory Park, announce two lantern-topped concrete pillars on either side of the entrance, each graced with a solemn maiden on a bronze placard. Monuments abound to honor the dead from that early 20th-century "war to end all wars" and those who fought and died in many conflicts since. There is a pond, a striking stone gazebo, a meditation chapel, and a reception center, the Memorial House. (The park is also a designated off-leash area for dogs.) Beyond the park wind a car-free paved road; a more rustic Freedom Trail following sinuous City Creek; and a haven for birds, animals, and people wishing to escape the nearby city's hubbub.

● Begin this walk on the northeast corner of the intersection where State St., North Temple and North Temple's eastern continuation, 2nd Ave., meet. An engraved boulder notes that this is City Creek Park. During much of the year, cool City Creek water flows under the rock bridge at the head of the trail, though that is not so in midwinter. Walk north, choosing one of several serpentine sidewalks, passing benches, a decorative bridge, and a seasonal drinking fountain. Glance down at the walkway and you'll spot the names of various local animals, often with images of their telltale tracks, from yellow-bellied marmot and white-tailed jackrabbit to bobcat and elk.

- After 0.14 mile, cross Canyon Rd. to the parklike center strip bordering a tamed and landscaped City Creek, and continue east. Here, in a spot now surrounded by venerable houses, once stood the Crismon Mill, the first gristmill built in the Territory of Utah, a marker notes.

- After another 0.1 mile, cross through the intersection of Fourth Ave. Off this dead-end side road are stairways that climb out of the canyon, to A St. on the east and lower Capitol Hill on the west.

- At 233 North, note quaint, redbrick Ottinger Hall, constructed in 1900 by the Volunteer Firemen's Association and used as a social hall and for other purposes for more than a century. A water chute on the west side of Canyon Rd. helps handle runoff and offers a pleasant gurgle.

- At 0.43 mile from the starting point, we reach the gate to Memory Grove, or Memory Park as it has been called. Here you have options: You can walk the paved road, where traffic is controlled and infrequent; choose the stone-paved sidewalks on either side; or follow the winding path on the park's east to see and contemplate the many war memorials. We recommend the latter.

- Half a mile into the walk is a marker introducing the Garden of Perception. Many plants, bushes, and trees are identified by signs of their own, including text in Braille. Here you can see, feel, and smell Andorra juniper, spreading yew, dwarf mugho pine, and more.

- Just beyond is a handsome World War I memorial, supported by stone pillars and known as the Pagoda. Marble used here came from the quarry in Vermont that supplied marble for the Lincoln Memorial in Washington, D.C. Lined with names of the lost, the Pagoda's text says it was dedicated in 1932 "in grateful remembrance of the heroic sons of Utah who gave their lives in the World War." To underline the solemn mood, a nearby flag and marker quote the lyrics of a song by Dorothy Alexander, a past president of Salt Lake City's Ladies Auxiliary of VFW Post 409, telling the dead, "The battle's o'er and peace is all around you. Sleep, soldier boy, sleep on."

- Next up, the Korean War of the early 1950s is remembered with a Wall of Honor. It sits above a City Creek retention pond, and across the canyon to the west are more sets of stairs and twin paths, which traverse Horizon Grove to Capitol Hill above.

- Also nearby are memorials honoring Utah's half-dozen Medal of Honor recipients, from World War II and the Vietnam War; a replica of the Liberty Bell across the pond; and a plaque and tree already noting the sacrifices of those who have served in conflicts in Iraq and Afghanistan.

- Like a small Greek temple, a pink marble Mediation Chapel rises at the foot of the canyon's eastern slope. Built in 1948 as a memorial to sons who died in World War II, it too offers poetry to set the scene in this peaceful place, calling upon the canyon breezes to comfort the dead: "Whate'er the season, canyon breeze, summer, autumn, winter, spring, the high adventure has been theirs: With gentle breath a requiem sing, to these, our sons, come home at rest."

- On the north side of the chapel are stones reminiscent of a cemetery, bearing names of those lost during battles at sea. An eagle-topped granite pillar and monument, "For God and Country," remembers the honored dead of the 145th U.S. Field Artillery.

- Across a bridge from these thought-provoking memorials sits an inviting building with deep-red doors and windbreaks. This is Memorial House. A marker tells us that this was actually a barn, toolhouse, and blacksmith shop for the city when it was built in 1904. As part of the Memory Park project, it was transformed in 1926 by the Service Star Legion into a social hall "in loving memory of

City Creek Canyon and Salt Lake City's skyline

those who gave their lives in defense of their country and of world freedom." Today it is often the site of wedding receptions.

- At the bridge, about 0.7 mile from the walk's start, are more choices: Many choose to walk the paved road up the canyon. Others follow the half-mile-long dirt Freedom Trail, which begins on the right side of the canyon and creek. The path itself has long existed, but it was improved, as a modern placard says, "to give people the opportunity to pause and ponder over the significant American liberties which they enjoy."

- The up-canyon walk offers another variety of peace. One mile from the start is a gate to further control canyon traffic. City Creek tumbles from mountains and hills far away. Small waterfalls sprinkle its course. A stairway, just after the trail begins, leads east and upward to Ninth Ave. In places are additional small war memorials. Additional bridges allow passage between the wooded path and the roadway, especially when Freedom Trail ends.

- Continue another half mile on the narrow paved road. Here lower City Creek Canyon ends at a junction where East Bonneville Blvd.—the one-way vehicular road from the city's Avenues neighborhood—meets West Bonneville Blvd., which continues one way (south) to the State Capitol. Here also is access to upper City Creek Canyon, a more extensive—and wild—option for walkers, joggers, cyclists, dogs, fishermen, and others. For this walk, however, veer left and loop west onto paved West Bonneville Blvd. The one-way road has a dedicated walk-bike path in its left lane and leads back to Capitol Hill.

- Walk an additional 0.9 mile south to connect with East Capitol Blvd. Along the way, the view of the city—the State Capitol, the Salt Lake City & County Building, and the Cathedral of the Madeleine are prominent on the skyline—opens as you emerge from City Creek Canyon. Deer and quail frequent the area. Geese can be heard cackling from a residence on City Creek's eastern slope.

- At 500 North, West Bonneville Blvd. ends. You are at the intersection with East Capitol Blvd., and the Capitol complex rises to the southwest. Veer onto a dirt path that parallels the paved road. After another 0.2 mile, head down one of the two sets of cement steps, first built by the Salt Lake Rotary Club in 1927, that descend into lower City Creek Canyon. The hillside paths were reconstructed in 2002.

● At the bottom of the steps, groomed Memory Grove again stretches before you. To complete this trek, turn right (south) and walk just over 0.4 mile to North Temple and City Creek Park, where the walk began

POINTS OF INTEREST (START TO FINISH)

Memory Grove 300 N. Canyon Rd.

Memorial House utahheritagefoundation.com/memorialhouse, 485 N. Canyon Rd.; 801-521-7969

Utah State Capitol utahstatecapitol.utah.gov, 350 N. State St.; 801-538-3074

ROUTE SUMMARY

1. Begin the walk at the northeast corner of State and North Temple Sts.
2. Enter City Creek Park and choose a northward route on various serpentine sidewalks, and then along Canyon Rd.
3. At about 0.4 mile, enter Memory Grove, a war-memorial park; continue north through the park.
4. After another 0.3 mile, either walk the mile-long dirt Freedom Trail on the east side of the canyon or remain on the paved road.
5. A gate, halting all vehicular traffic in lower City Creek Canyon, is located 1 mile from the start. Walk up City Creek another 0.7 mile to the intersection of West Bonneville and East Bonneville Blvds., both one-way auto routes, traveling east to west.
6. Veer left and loop west onto West Bonneville Blvd., which has a dedicated walk-bike path.
7. Walk 0.9 mile to connect with East Capitol Blvd., northeast of the State Capitol.
8. At this junction, veer left onto a dirt path that parallels the paved road.
9. Continue another 0.2 mile and descend either of two cement stairways and paths that lead into City Creek Canyon.
10. At the bottom of the steps, turn right and walk south through lower Memory Grove.
11. Continue down the canyon just over 0.4 mile to North Temple and State Sts., where the walk began.

CONNECTING THE WALKS

Two western stairways out of Memory Grove connect with Walk 6, Capitol Hill. The City Creek Canyon and Capitol Hill walks also connect at East Capitol Blvd., if you veer west and do not descend back into City Creek Canyon and Memory Grove, near the end of this walk.

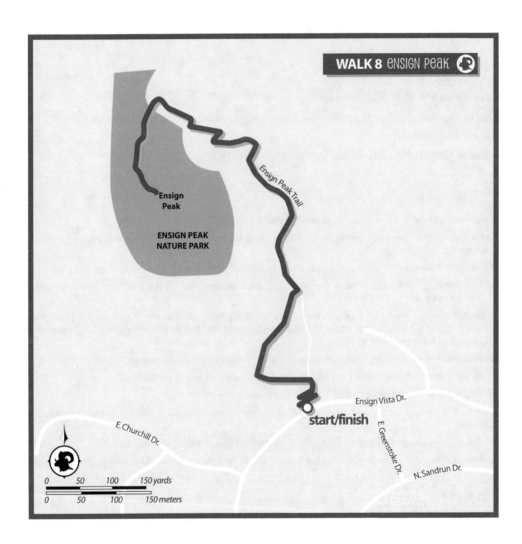

WALK 8 ENSIGN PEAK

Ensign Peak Trail

Ensign
Peak

ENSIGN PEAK
NATURE PARK

Ensign Vista Dr.

start/finish

E. Churchill Dr.

E. Greenstoke Dr.

N. Sandrun Dr.

0   50   100   150 yards
0   50   100   150 meters

8 ENSIGN PEAK: SACRED SUMMIT WITH A HEAVENLY VIEW

BOUNDARIES: **Ensign Vista Dr., Churchill Dr., Sandhurst Dr., Meridian Peak (Wasatch Mountain foothills)**
DISTANCE: **1.2 miles (round-trip)**
DIFFICULTY: **Strenuous**
PARKING: **Limited free street parking on Ensign Vista Dr.**
PUBLIC TRANSIT: **None**

If Salt Lake City has a "sacred mountain"—something akin, perhaps, to Mounts Fuji, Olympus, and Sinai—then Ensign Peak fills the bill. It lacks the height or craggy majesty of those revered prominences, but no other summit can match its significance in Utah's pioneer and religious history. As a bonus, the vantage offers a splendid view of the Salt Lake Valley: The metropolitan area spreads southward like a 3-D map at your feet: streets, buildings, fields, and trees, with the Wasatch and Oquirrh ranges enfolding the panoramic view like great, often snow-dappled parentheses.

Ensign Peak derives its importance from Brigham Young. The American Moses, who led pioneers to the Salt Lake Valley in 1847, told of a vision he experienced in the Mormon temple in Nauvoo, Illinois, which members of The Church of Jesus Christ of Latter-day Saints were obliged to flee following the murder of founder Joseph Smith. Early church leader George A. Smith, in an 1869 address, told the story. In the vision, he said, Joseph Smith showed Brigham Young "the mountain that we now call Ensign Peak, immediately north of Salt Lake City, and there was an ensign (that) fell upon that peak, and Joseph said, 'Build under that point where the colors fall, and you will prosper and have peace.'"

Today it is the high centerpiece of Ensign Peak Nature Park, a joint project of the Ensign Peak Foundation and the city. A landscaped plaza, completed in 1996, is surrounded by several informational and historical markers. Also accessible to the handicapped, the plaza serves as the park's entrance and trailhead. Paths sprout to nearby Vista Mound, just above, and to the top of Ensign Peak itself. The latter, beyond the landscaped area, is more of a rugged little hike than a leisurely walk on a city street; the elevation gain is 398 feet, steep in places, and ragged from erosion and use. The short trek is nevertheless a favorite of families and groups, as well as solo hikers—and most will agree that the reward is worth it.

The capitol is visible below, in the near distance, and downtown Salt Lake City lies beyond that. The views of the industrial Beck St. area, Salt Lake City International Airport, and the Great Salt Lake to the west are spectacular. People hike the trail in all seasons, even in snow or mud, as telltale footprints reveal. With wildflowers in bloom and moderate temperatures, late spring and early summer are fine times to hike Ensign. In midsummer the trek is best done early or at sunset (a popular hour). Be aware of the weather (lightning storms can move in quickly), and bringing water along is always a good idea, even though the route to Ensign Peak's summit is only about a mile round-trip.

- Begin your hike at Ensign Peak Nature Park, 1002 N. Ensign Vista Dr., which is about a mile and a half north of downtown Salt Lake City's North Temple. To get to the starting point, go north up State St. to its head, in front of the Utah State Capitol. Turn right (east) onto East Capitol Blvd., which curves around the statehouse's east side. Continue uphill north into the Ensign Downs residential neighborhood. Turn left (west) onto Ensign Vista Dr. (about 1000 North). Ensign Peak Nature Park and the trailhead are directly above the Ensign Peak LDS Ward meetinghouse, just beyond Greenstoke Dr. Across Ensign Vista Dr. is peaceful, Mormon-oriented Ensign Peak Memorial Garden, a pioneer sesquicentennial garden project of the area's LDS congregations.

- Enter the park's plaza, on the street's north side, which has both stairways and an inclined sidewalk ramp. A concrete wall encircles a brick world map at your feet. Markers and maps lining the wall include the original 1934 historical plaque from Ensign Peak's summit that was stolen and lost for decades. It tells of a trek by Brigham Young and other pioneers only days after their arrival in the Salt Lake Valley in 1847, at which time they "made a careful survey of the mountains, canyons, and streams." Other placards note the earlier presence in the valley, or nearby, of Indians and explorers and offer details about nature in the region, from food sources like pine nuts and wild raspberries to insect life and mammals.

- Go to the plaza's east side, turn left (north), and follow signs along the well-marked trail. The first portion of the trail is concrete, making it wheelchair-accessible.

- At an intersection in the paved pathway, just above the plaza, turn left (west) onto a concrete tributary path, about 300 feet long, leading to Vista Mound, low on the peak's south side. The view here is excellent, if not quite equal to that on the top of Ensign Peak. An illustrated marker offers a quick study of the valley beyond: the Wasatch Mountains, the University of Utah, the State Capitol building, city hall (the Salt Lake City & County Building), and Kennecott's open-pit copper mine in the Oquirrh Mountains.

- Turn around to continue up the hillside. A thin fence-line trail heading north from Vista Mound connects to the main Ensign Peak trail, which can also be accessed if you return along the paved walkway to where the short Vista Mound path first diverged. If you follow the latter course, turn left (north) at the junction, and proceed along the main trail, which soon is no longer paved. A small sitting area with several concrete-block "seats" is near where the trail north from Vista Mound and the principal peak trail converge.

- Follow the well-worn, erosion-furrowed dirt trail uphill, as it proceeds in a traversing zigzag up the back of Ensign Peak. Fences, stones, fallen tree trunks, and warning signs attempt to keep hikers on the trail and out of reclamation areas to allow the hillside to heal from decades of abuse. One trailside marker at a potential rest area presents an old-style map of the valley, while text describes the rise of the mountain ranges and describes the valley below.

- The trail steepens as it rises toward a ridge on the west. Here, again, is a good spot for a break—this one offering a view to the west, over Salt Lake's industrial northwest, the airport, and the Great Salt Lake. A marker (often spray-painted by vandals, as is unfortunately common on

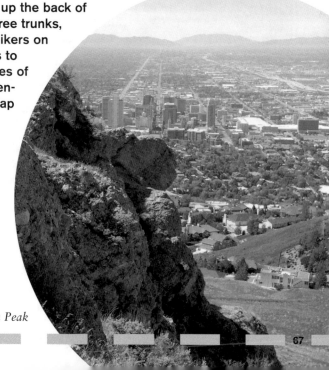

A view from Ensign Peak

Back Story

Brigham Young, who had been ill, entered the Salt Lake Valley on Saturday, July 24, 1847. Other Mormon pioneers had arrived in the two preceding days. They spent all of the next day, Sunday, resting and worshiping. However, on July 26, one of the first tasks attempted by a small party of men, including Brigham Young, was to climb what is now known as Ensign Peak to get a better look at the valley. It was also a chance to see firsthand a mountain Brigham Young had seen in a vision in faraway Nauvoo, Illinois, one in which his assassinated predecessor, Joseph Smith, told him of a peak below which his followers could peaceably settle in the West.

On the summit in 1847, we are told, Brigham Young said, "Here is a proper place to raise an ensign to the nations," a Biblical reference. According to a 1934 historical marker, Wilford Woodruff, later a president of The Church of Jesus Christ of Latter-day Saints, was the first to ascend, and he "suggested it as a fitting place to 'set up an ensign' (Isaiah 11:12). It was then named Ensign Peak."

The 1934 historical marker also notes that subsequently "the stars and stripes were raised here"—though that undoubtedly came later, researchers say. Flags, especially U.S. flags, have become particularly linked to Ensign Peak. The American flag was flown from a special flagpole on Ensign Peak on July 24, 1897, complete with a 21-gun salute, in commemoration of the 50th anniversary of the pioneers' arrival. Utah had become a state a year earlier, in 1896. A similar celebration was held on Ensign Peak in 1947, the pioneer centennial.

Not long after the pioneers settled in the Salt Lake Valley, Ensign Peak also "became sacred to many as a place for meditation," notes one Ensign Peak Nature Park marker. "Prior to completion of [the Salt Lake LDS Temple], religious ordinances were performed" by pioneers, probably on the hillside. It was, in essence, an outdoor temple—a sacred mountain.

Ensign's signs) tells the story of both the salt-laden contemporary lake below and its prehistoric precursor, Lake Bonneville. In spring, flowers speckle the hillside here, from tiny phlox to crimson Indian paintbrush, usually seen in alpine settings.

- If you have paused, continue uphill to the south, toward Ensign Peak's summit. The trail, bordered by giant boulders that look like ancient concrete, gets rockier, serpentine, and more exposed, as the western slope is very clifflike. Keep a close eye on children, if they're along for the hike. In some places, fences help keep trekkers safe.

- On Ensign Peak's top, 5,416 feet above sea level, is a towering stone monument with an oval cap. On the pillar's south side is the 1934 historical marker, a later duplicate of the one on the streetside plaza below. A half dozen modern placards outline Ensign Peak's history and significance and pinpoint valley landmarks. The 18-foot-tall summit monument and marker were built and placed here on July 26, 1934, by the Salt Lake Ensign Stake Mutual Improvement Association. Stones gathered all along the Mormon Trail, from Illinois to Utah, are incorporated into the monument.

- Return to this route's start via the same zigzagging trail, back to the Ensign Peak Nature Park plaza and Ensign Vista Dr.

POINTS OF INTEREST (START TO FINISH)

Ensign Peak Nature Park 1002 N. Ensign Vista Dr.

Ensign Downs Park 125 E. Dorchester Dr.

Ensign Peak Memorial Garden about 1000 N. Ensign Vista Dr.

ROUTE SUMMARY

1. Begin your hike at the Ensign Peak Nature Park, 1002 N. Ensign Vista Dr.
2. Visit Ensign Peak Nature Park's plaza. On the plaza's east side is a paved path.
3. Follow the concrete path to a junction. Turn left (west) to Vista Mound.
4. Continue uphill via a short dirt trail heading north from Vista Mound, or return to the paved path's trail intersection and turn left (north) to Ensign Peak's main dirt trail.
5. Continue uphill as the trail traverses the peak's north side to the summit.
6. On top are a stone monument, additional markers, and a protective metal railing.
7. Reverse the route to return to the park's plaza and Ensign Vista Dr.

CONNECTING THE WALKS

Connect with Walk 2, Capitol Hill, 1 mile south on East Capitol Blvd.

Connect with Walk 3, Memory Grove/City Creek Canyon, 1 mile south on East Capitol Blvd.

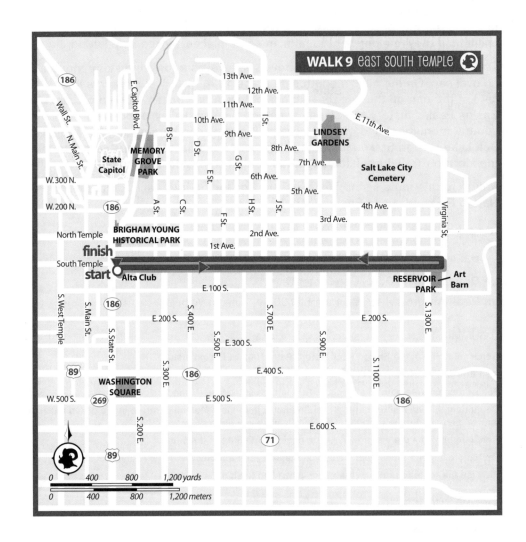

WALK 9 east south temple

186

Wall St.

N. Main St.

E. Capitol Blvd.

B St.

D St.

E St.

F St.

G St.

H St.

1 St.

J St.

13th Ave.

12th Ave.

11th Ave.

10th Ave.

9th Ave.

8th Ave.

7th Ave.

6th Ave.

5th Ave.

4th Ave.

3rd Ave.

2nd Ave.

1st Ave.

E. 11th Ave.

LINDSEY GARDENS

Salt Lake City Cemetery

Virginia St.

State Capitol

MEMORY GROVE PARK

W. 300 N.

W. 200 N.

186

A St.

C St.

North Temple

BRIGHAM YOUNG HISTORICAL PARK

finish

South Temple

start   Alta Club

RESERVOIR PARK

Art Barn

S. West Temple

S. Main St.

S. State St.

186

E. 100 S.

S. 400 E.

S. 500 E.

S. 700 E.

S. 900 E.

S. 1100 E.

S. 1300 E.

E. 200 S.

E. 200 S.

E. 300 S.

89

S. 300 E.

186

E. 400 S.

WASHINGTON SQUARE

W. 500 S.

269

E. 500 S.

186

S. 200 E.

E. 600 S.

89

71

0   400   800   1,200 yards

0   400   800   1,200 meters

9 east SOUTH TeMPLe: TIMe TraveLING ON 'BrIGHaM STreeT'

BOUNDARIES: **South Temple, from State St. to Virginia St./University St.**
DISTANCE: **3 miles**
DIFFICULTY: **Easy**
PARKING: **Metered parking on most streets, free street parking the farther east you park; underground parking at the Joseph Smith Memorial Building (15 E. South Temple)**
PUBLIC TRANSIT: **The downtown TRAX light-rail station is a block and a half away from this walk's start, at 50 S. Main St. Many buses go up and down State St. Bus #6 makes regular stops along South Temple, should you get tired, but exact fare is required.**

Although properly known as South Temple, for many in the late 19th and early 20th centuries, this was Brigham St. It slopes gently from pioneer leader Brigham Young's Beehive House and Eagle Gate at State St. toward Salt Lake City's eastern benches. Here civic leaders, mining magnates, bankers, and other businessmen and businesswomen built dozens of mansions. Some were grand, even grandiose, others more modest—and a great number survive to this day. Ironically, many of their residents were Gentiles, as early Mormons called those not of their faith, and therefore not followers of Brother Brigham, though they lived on "his" street. Here, too, are architectural treasures such as the city's premier Catholic church, the Cathedral of the Madeleine; First Presbyterian Church; and the Salt Lake Masonic Temple. A hundred years ago, as Margaret D. Lester notes in her pictorial history, *Brigham Street,* this prestigious boulevard "became the most beautiful thoroughfare between Denver and San Francisco."

South Temple is a route worthy of the word *promenade.* A wide, recently rebuilt and repaved street, it is lined with mature shade trees. Carriage stepping-stones and bridle posts still sit curbside in front of a few yards. Salt Lake City declared the upscale neighborhood to be its first official historic district in 1975. According to material nominating the stretch to the National Register of Historic Places, "South Temple is significant as the first stately residential boulevard in Utah, and remains today, much of it still residential, as a reminder of a lifestyle that is gone." Indeed, in 1982, South Temple was named a National Historic District. More recently, South Temple was honored by the American Planning Association as one of America's 10 great streets.

The historic district spans the 1.5 miles between State St., on the west, and Virginia St./ University St. (1350 East), on the east. On the street's south side are 10½ standard—and therefore long—central-city blocks. The north side is the fringe of Salt Lake City's nonstandard, hillside Avenues neighborhood, which has 20 small blocks. At eight standard blocks to the mile, it is easy to determine how far you will go on this route, since the suggested return is on the south side of South Temple.

Today, as many commercial enterprises as homes line the street, with many businesses occupying what once were opulent residences. The walk is gradually uphill, more so the final five blocks eastward. Many houses and other structures bear placards noting that they are on the National Register, but of course we can't describe all of the 136 historic buildings here. In brief, the architectural range is remarkable: from Classical Revival, Queen Anne, and Prairie-style houses and mansions to the Victorian Romanesque rigor of the Cathedral of the Madeleine and the Egyptian Revival majesty of the Masonic Temple. The Utah Heritage Foundation recommends taking 2½ hours to tour the area. You can begin the walk on either side of the street, but we're recommending a tree-shaded stroll on the north side first. Street signs will note your progress through the alphabet (A St., B St., etc., on the north) and hundreds (200 East, 300 East, etc., on the south), but note that street names and numbers are also stamped in most sidewalks.

● **Begin the walk on the southeast corner of State St. and South Temple, beside the Alta Club building. The gentlemen's club was founded in 1883, named after the wealth-generating town and mining district at the top of nearby Little Cottonwood Canyon by mining magnates and businessmen—none of them Mormons, who were excluded. Mormon/non-Mormon divisions ran deep at the time, in business, in politics, in the newspapers, and personally, so it is interesting to think of this anti-Mormon haven sitting kitty-corner to the stately residence of Brother Brigham, as Brigham Young was generally called at the time by his flock. The blocky four-story Alta Club, which opened in 1898, showcases the Second Renaissance Revival style. For nearly a century, women were not allowed to join the club, either, though apparently wives were welcome. A successful antidiscrimination lawsuit in 1987 finally opened the club to nonwidowed women. The structure was renovated in a $4 million project in 2001.**

● At the intersection, cross to South Temple's north side and begin strolling east. The Eagle Gate Apartments on the intersection's northeast corner have the look of another era, but the buildings are actually modern structures, built to replace tattered predecessors with the same name. The first historic structure then, next door to the east, is the Elks Club Building. The fraternal Benevolent and Protective Order of Elks moved out a few decades ago. Their 1923 clubhouse was remodeled for professional offices. A large complex—the Brigham Condominiums—is the new neighbor to the east, joining a historic multifamily apartment campus on A St., the Covey and Buckingham apartment buildings. These were constructed just over a century ago, in 1909.

● *Majestic, moody,* and *medieval* describe the Gothic Revival edifice that is Salt Lake City's Cathedral of the Madeleine, built from 1899 to 1909—glance up to the towers and you'll glimpse nasty-looking gargoyles protruding high overhead. Refurbished during the 1990s in an effort involving much of the community, the Catholic cathedral's interior is bathed in soft stained-glass light, which falls upon rows of pews, carved wooden altarpieces, and beautiful murals. The cornerstone offers a slightly different name for this landmark: "St. Mary's Cathedral," it says. "Erected A.D. 1900." A plaque noting that the edifice is on the National Register of Historic Places, however, reads: "Cathedral of the Madeleine. Begun with land purchase in 1889. Dedicated 1909. Architects: C. M. Neuhausen, B. O. Mecklenburg, John Comes. Built under leadership of Bishop Lawrence Scanlan with monies from the Pius Fund, mining philanthropists, and parishioners." Catholic diocese offices are to the northeast on this all-Catholic block.

First Presbyterian Church

● Continue to C St. and you will come upon a church that looks as if it has been transported intact from the British Isles. First Presbyterian Church was built from 1903 to 1906 of creamy salmon sandstone quarried in Red Butte Canyon, east of the city. The church boasts a crenellated square tower and lancet-shaped stained-glass windows depicting Christ in the manger, at Gethsemane, and at the first Easter. These are, the Utah Heritage Foundation declares, artistic treasures. The sanctuary's acoustics are excellent, and the church hosts many concerts and cultural events.

● As fortunes declined, families scattered, and houses aged in the mid-20th century, several of South Temple's venerable homes and gilded mansions fell on hard times. Many simply fell…to wrecking crews. The homes of some of Utah's biggest bigwigs—businessman-builder Samuel Newhouse, inventor Philo T. Farnsworth (television!), Governor George Dern—were demolished. As you'll see, shops, offices, and even filling stations took their place. The palatial home of Western mining entrepreneur Enos A. Wall and his wife, Mary, at 411 E. South Temple, however, had a different fate: It became a Jewish center, an insurance company, and ultimately a school, LDS Business College. Though the college recently moved, the column-lined portico and overall grace of the villalike Wall manse still sit at the heart of the estate turned campus, classroom extensions bracketing it on either side.

● Just to the east, where the Avenues' E St. and midtown's 500 East almost align, service stations, stores, and diners popped up in what became a mini–business district on South Temple. Although fewer in number today, such establishments continue to thrive. For instance, if you are in need of refreshment, a snack, or a meal, an Einstein Bros bagel shop and The Wild Grape Bistro occupy one north-side corner. The venerable Pagoda restaurant, offering Japanese fare, sits just behind them on E St.

● Continuing east, truly impressive residences (and ex-residences) adorn Brigham St. and its tree-lined northern sidewalk. On the east corner of F St., at 529 E. South Temple, is one of the loveliest: the creamy, neoclassical Keith mansion. David Keith, in tandem with friend Thomas Kearns, whose palace is just up the street, earned his riches in Park City's silver mines. He became a merchant (Salt Lake's vanished Keith-O'Brien department store), builder, and banker. The grand home he and his wife, Mary, built was transformed into an elegant business building, with a rotunda and a stained-glass skylight. An impressive carriage house, to the side, once included a bowling alley, a shooting gallery, and servants quarters. East of the Keith mansion, neighboring residences serve as offices.

● One of the history-packed crown jewels of South Temple rises on the east corner of G St., a residence that is today the Utah Governor's Mansion. This chateau—for that is what it is, an out-of-place replica mimicking the French renaissance—was built in 1900 by soon-to-be U.S. Senator Thomas Kearns and his wife, Jennie. With an exterior of light-toned oolitic limestone from central Utah, the mansion's interior is filled with fine mahogany and oak woodwork and marble tiles. Take note of the stone carriage step, still in place on the South Temple curb. Partnered with David Keith, Kearns made his fortune in Park City's silver mines, but he was more than a miner: He built the stately Kearns Building on Main St.; served a term as a U.S. senator, from 1901 to 1905; was co-owner of *The Salt Lake Tribune*; and, unfortunately, was an early automobile fatality, struck by a car at Main St. and South Temple in 1918. In 1937 the Kearns family donated the great house to the state. Utah's gubernatorial families lived here until 1957. For the next 23 years the mansion was home to the Utah Historical Society. After extensive renovation, the governor and his family returned in 1980. Unfortunately, a quick-moving Christmastime fire in 1993 seared much of the mansion's interior woodwork. Another ambitious project restored the residence to its former glory. You can ogle the interior beauty for yourself: Tours are offered seasonally in June, July, August, and early December, on Tuesdays and Thursdays, 2–4 p.m.

● The Epley/Glendinning House, at 617 E. South Temple, is a former residence that draws from varied architectural styles, from Italianate to Victorian. Its appearance does, however, justify the word *antique.* Built by a mining engineer in 1883, it subsequently was the home of James Glendinning, an alcoholic and financially troubled Salt Lake City mayor, Utah Heritage Foundation historians say. In 1898 the Glendinnings lost the home during a foreclosure. (Sound familiar?) Today it is the home of the Utah Arts Council. The nearby, turreted Kahn mansion, at 678 E. South Temple, was built by a family of Jewish grocers.

● Cross I St., a major north-south Avenues artery. Even-busier 700 East is askew across South Temple, so watchfully negotiate this complicated intersection. A great many homes that once decorated the next several blocks have been erased for more prosaic enterprises: office buildings, medical facilities, apartments, and gas stations. In contrast, at the head of 700 East, Busath Photography has maintained the evocative elegance and landscaping of the Evans House, a Tudor-style home built in 1911.

- At 731 E. South Temple is the relatively tame Sherman/Jackling House, a Colonial-inspired residence from 1898. Its most colorful resident was probably Daniel Jackling, an engineer whose mass-production methods for processing low-grade copper ore revolutionized the industry. His most visible legacy: the mountain-chewing open-pit Kennecott Copper Mine, one of the largest in the world, visible along the Oquirrh range on the Salt Lake Valley's southwest edge. In her book *Brigham Street,* Margaret D. Lester says Jackling was described as "the greatest of the greats." He was, she observes, both a hardworking genius and a playboy who maintained multiple mistresses. Rich as Croesus, Jackling didn't reside on South Temple for long. He lived in hotel suites in Salt Lake City and San Francisco for the rest of his life.

- On the brink of L St., at 839 E. South Temple, are the Maryland Apartments, a century-old complex with an ornamented exterior, including balconies with balustrades and substantial columns supporting the front portico. It was designed and built by Salt Lake architect Bernard O. Mecklenburg, who also lived here. Read a few of the National Historic District placards on the houses along East South Temple and you might come to the conclusion that the thoroughfare should be called Mecklenburg-Neuhausen St. (for Mecklenburg and the appropriately surnamed Carl M. Neuhausen), not Brigham St. They were the primary designers of the Cathedral of the Madeleine, as well.

- At 935 E. South Temple is a modern Ronald McDonald House, for ill children and their families. Farther east, fresh uses have been found for several historic-district homes. The porch-wrapped Filer House, a 1904 residence at 943 E. South Temple, has been transformed into Haxton Manor, a Victorian-style bed-and-breakfast. The Wrigley house, at 973 E. South Temple, stands out because of its modern, Spanish Colonial Revival style, featuring stucco walls, arched windows and entries, and stained glass. The redbrick house with green columns, white trim, and a big porch at 1037 E. South Temple is actually Lyon & Healy West Harpmasters, a showroom for harps, harp accessories, and music. The Town Club, an elite civic, social, and charitable organization for women, has occupied the handsome brick residence at 1081 E. South Temple since 1939. The home was built in 1906 by Frances Walker, the widow of Samuel Walker. He was one of four prominent merchant-banker brothers. Today it, too, is trimmed in white, a patriotic flagpole standing at attention in the yard. At 1135 E. South Temple is a second Ronald McDonald House Charities site. Merchant Walter Lyne and his wife, Alice, built the Victorian mansion in 1898. More recently, it was the Brigham Street Inn, a bed-and-breakfast that was sold to the charity in 2004.

● Continue east to R St. On one corner you can't help but notice the sheltered entrance to a subterranean walkway. Wasatch Elementary School sits on South Temple's north side, but the playground is on the south side. In 1931 a tunnel was carved under the busy avenue to safeguard schoolchildren as they made their way between the two locations. The tunnel's entryways often sport colorful paper decorations encouraging the children and school spirit.

● As the sidewalk's grade steepens toward 1350 E. South Temple, the eclectic architecture—and sometimes quirky landscaping—continues. At 1167 E. South Temple sits one of the street's classic red-brick homes, this one with a distinctive black border. The striking 1912 Armstrong residence, its classic, columned portico giving it the appearance of an antebellum Southern mansion, occupies 1177 E. South Temple. It is believed to have been designed by Richard K. A. Kletting, architect of Utah's statehouse. A shingled 1895 home with a single cone-topped turret at 1205 E. South Temple, on the other hand, looks like it would be at home on Cape Cod. In 1905 it was purchased by Joseph Walker Jr. and his wife, Margaret, more members of the prominent Utah merchant and banking family. A tempting iron-bench sculpture— street furniture at its finest—might puzzle passersby outside the elegant

The Kearns Mansion, Utah's Governor's Residence

Back Story

During the 19th century, South Temple was a dusty, dirty, rutted, and sometimes boggy path. It was the primary route between Salt Lake City and its foothills, the mountains, and the U.S. military's Fort Douglas. The street bustled with horses, carriages, and wagons carrying goods, timber, and quarried stone. A slaughter-house stood on its eastern end, says the Utah Heritage Foundation's online guide, **UtahHeritageFoundation.com.** Not until 1903 was it paved; mud and slush gave way to automobiles and trolley cars.

Great sycamores, as well as pine, spruce, ash, and oak trees, line South Temple today, most of them planted a century ago. So do mansions—ranging from the grace-ful to the pretentious—built by wealthy mine owners, speculators, and merchants. It was, at its peak, an enchanting place to live, Margaret D. Lester wrote in *Brigham Street,* her history of the nicknamed avenue. The wealthy were neighbors to the rich, and parties, teas, fancy balls, and lavish weddings spiced the scene. After the turn of the 20th century, South Temple was a favorite for those out for a Sunday stroll—just as it still can be.

By the 1960s, the ambience, safety, and captivating history of South Temple gal-vanized preservationists and city leaders to try to halt or limit the destruction of its past. In 1975, Salt Lake City declared South Temple its first historic district. That preservation effort continued, and in 1982 it was placed on the National Register as the South Temple Historic District. Mansions and cottages, apart-ments and condominiums, office buildings and shops contribute to its modern mix. Today's South Temple retains both its glory and its charm.

Colonial Revival mansion at 1229 E. South Temple. One could get the impression that Charlie Chaplin had dropped by, absentmindedly forgetting his derby and umbrella—except they are metal and attached to the bench. Appropriately, or perhaps coinciden-tally, the house was first owned by Louis Terry, who ran a furniture store.

● Climb with care the short sidewalk staircase just beyond the Federal Heights Apartments (built in 1930 in the Federal Revival style, of course) at 1321 E. South Temple. Before you is Virginia St., and your walk through the Avenues alphabet is complete. On the other side of South Temple, on the same alignment as Virginia, is University St.; the University of Utah is nearby. At this four-way stop, cross right, to the south side of South Temple, and then turn right again to begin your downhill return to the west.

- Salt Lake City's Reservoir Park occupies the block to your right. It includes grassy play areas, picnic tables, a playground, and an art gallery. In the park's center is The Art Barn, home of the Salt Lake City Arts Council and Finch Lane Galley. Yes, until recently there was an underground reservoir here. The 1300 East Reservoir was built on the block's southwest corner in 1901. In 1956 the reservoir was covered and tennis courts were built on the concrete surface. After a partial collapse in 2009, the reservoir was decommissioned and demolished, except for an antique wall and lampposts fronting 1300 East, a major north-south traffic corridor.

- Across from R St. is the southern entrance to the pedestrian tunnel that allows safe passage for students from Wasatch Elementary School to and from their playground, which is here on South Temple's south side. Several smaller residences on the block between 1300 East and 1200 East have been turned into the Kanzeon Zen Center of Utah.

- Although there are grand mansions on the south side of South Temple, many homes along this part of the route generally would be deemed more modest. In an online tour guide, the Utah Heritage Foundation points to the Ayres homes at 1264 and 1266 E. South Temple, observing, "Many prosperous Salt Lake City businessmen built homes on South Temple hoping to share in the prestige of their wealthy neighbors." The Ayres were upper middle class, and apparently built homes here as investments, for they quickly sold them. At 1106 and 1108 E. South Temple are two redbrick residences dating to 1901 and 1908, the Patrick Moran House and Cottage. It may be worthwhile to look down: The grainy, century-old concrete beneath your feet on much of this route may well be part of Moran's legacy; his crews poured concrete for many a sidewalk and curb, as well as major water conduits, while modernizing Salt Lake City.

- The Salt Lake Regional Medical Center—known through most of its history as Holy Cross Hospital, a Catholic institution—is today a hodgepodge of medical buildings old and new occupying the block between 1100 East and 1000 East. The hospital was founded in 1875 in much smaller quarters by the Sisters of the Holy Cross of St. Bartholomew, with volunteer doctors. This site's main building went up from 1881 to 1883. Several additions were made early in the 20th century (with architectural contributions from none other than Brigham St. architecture veterans Carl M. Neuhausen and Bernard O. Mecklenburg). Major reconstruction has continued, as the hospital remains one of urban Salt Lake City's principal medical facilities. The early hospital's stoic Holy Cross Chapel, dedicated in 1904, is visible from South Temple amid scores of vehicles and steel-and-glass modernity.

- Farther along, at 974 E. South Temple, is the Frank Cameron House, which sports a variety of masonry patterns. Built in 1908, its real claim to fame dates to 1929, when heavyweight boxing champion Jack Dempsey purchased the home for his mother. The hard-punching Dempsey—renowned as "The Manassa Mauler" (he was from Manassa, Colorado)—lived and trained in Salt Lake City for part of his epic career. The Haven, a substance abuse treatment center, now occupies the residence.

- At 940 E. South Temple, introduced by sandstone pillars topped by ribbonlike ironwork arches, is one of the historic district's anomalies: Haxton Place, a cul-de-sac lined with nine substantial homes. The tiny subneighborhood was established in 1909. Among the first residents were the nook's developers, James Keith and Thomas Griffin. Haxton Place is named for a street in London, from which Griffin hailed, the Utah Heritage Foundation tells us.

- The stolid brick structure at 850 E. South Temple has a Prairie-style/Frank Lloyd Wright look about it, as it nestles nicely into the historic neighborhood. Yet this is not a residence; it is, and has been since it was built in 1912, the Ladies Literary Club. The club was founded to promote libraries in Utah and remains active today. People and organizations can rent its ballroom and other facilities. The Shingle style emerges at the George Downey House, at 808 E. South Temple. The 1893 residence has been transformed into modern law offices, but an ages-old mining cart out front reminds passersby of the site's mining legacy.

- Pass the parking lot for Bryant Junior High School, which is on the other side of the block, and a burnt-red Thai restaurant, Sawadee, at 754 E. South Temple. Then it is

time to navigate 700 East, at its busy intersection with South Temple, further complicated by the current of cars coming from and going to the Avenues' I St. The north-
south I St. and 700 East are not precisely aligned, so be aware of the traffic patterns.

- The wood-trimmed, redbrick, and turreted Queen Anne–style home on the southwest
corner at 678 E. South Temple was built for Jewish-immigrant merchants Emanuel
and Fanny Kahn. Today it is the Anniversary Inn, a bed-and-breakfast. For contrast, the
stately Masonic Temple hulks next door, at 650 E. South Temple. Constructed in 1927,
the temple is considered the city's best example of Egyptian Revival architecture. A
pair of half-man, half-lion sphinxes, each protecting a dark globe between its ample
paws, dominate the front staircase. Tours of the temple are available, by arrangement,
on Tuesday and Thursday afternoons.

- Residential elegance on a massive scale is evident at 610 E. South Temple, filled
by the Second Renaissance Revival–style Walker-McCarthey Mansion. It was built in
1904 for Matthew and Angelena Walker. Walker was the youngest of four brothers
who immigrated to Utah in 1849. They began selling merchandise to settlers and the
Army, and their store evolved into Walker Bank, one of Utah's fabled financial institutions. According to a large plaque outside, the Walkers' vast (18,700 square feet)
and ornate mansion was purchased in 1999 and restored by businessman Philip G.
McCarthey. Beware: Stone lions guard its front entry.

- The delicate-looking Gentsch-Thompson home, on 600 East's western corner, is
another eye-catching antique, built in 1889 in the Victorian Eclectic style. Like several
other residences along South Temple, this was the home of a mayor: Ezra Thompson
was in office for three terms, beginning in 1899. He and his family later moved into
the Keith Mansion, across the street to the west. Farther west you will pass a nearly
block-wide modern condominium-office complex. Inside, unheralded by any signage,
are the national offices of the Sinclair Oil Co.

- Cross the busy confluence of 500 East and South Temple. The Avenues' E St. is again
across the way. Several lots are empty, convenience stories and apartment buildings
having disappeared over the past few decades. But at 430 E. South Temple is a building that once housed A.O. Whitmore Electric Automobiles, a firm that operated from
1910 to 1920. (Doesn't the resurgence of electric cars add just a touch of irony?)

The wide building is now subdivided and houses a variety of businesses, including a bridal shop, an art framing and design firm, the Black Sheep Wool Co. (a yarn craft shop), and Mrs. Backers Pastry Shop. You might want to step inside the bakery to sample the sweet atmosphere, examine the extravagant wedding cakes, and perhaps purchase a fruit-filled tart or a few of the cupcakes topped by the bakery's signature sugar blossoms. They are so pretty it seems a shame to eat them.

● As you head west on South Temple toward downtown, historic houses become rare, as shops, outlets, and offices take precedence. Those homes that survive have been repurposed. At 260 E. South Temple is the Hagensbarth house, now Larkin Mortuary. Built in 1914, it has been a funeral home since 1925. The simple (for South Temple) Heber J. Grant house was built in 1904 at 174 E. South Temple. Grant, a financial leader, was president of The Church of Jesus Christ of Latter-day Saints during the Great Depression. The small, European-style, brick Carlton Hotel Inn & Suites, built at 140 E. South Temple in the 1920s, snuggles up to the skyscraping University Club Building. At street level is a small sandwich shop, Skool Lunch, which might be a comfortable stop for refreshment or a meal. Just beyond is the corner Alta Club, front flags waving, where your promenade along this ritzy Salt Lake City thorough-fare began.

POINTS OF INTEREST (START TO FINISH)

Cathedral of the Madeleine, saltlakecathedral.org, 331 E. South Temple, 801-328-8941

First Presbyterian Church of Salt Lake fpcslc.org, 12 C St., 801-363-3889

Pagoda pagodaslc.com, 26 E St., 801-355-8155

Utah Governor's Mansion utah.gov/governor/mansion, 603 E. South Temple, 801-538-1005

Haxton Manor haxtonmanor.com, 943 E. South Temple, 877-930-4646

The Art Barn in Reservoir Park (Salt Lake City Arts Council) slcclassic.com/arts/pages/artbarn2.htm, 1340 E. South Temple, 801-596-5000

Sawadee sawadee1.com, 754 E. South Temple, 801-328-8424

Anniversary Inn anniversaryinn.com/south-temple, 678 E. South Temple, 800-363-4960

Salt Lake Masonic Temple wasatchlodge.org, 650 E. South Temple, 801-363-2936

Mrs. Backers Pastry Shop mrsbackers.com, 434 E. South Temple, 801-532-2022

Carlton Hotel Inn & Suites carltonhotel-slc.com, 140 E. South Temple, 800-633-3500

Skool Lunch Deli & Bakery 136 E. South Temple, 801-532-5269, southtemple@skoollunch.com

route summary

1. Begin at the southeast corner of State St. and South Temple, outside the Alta Club building.
2. Cross to the north side of South Temple.
3. Turn east and stroll this simple east-west route to Virginia St. (1350 E. South Temple), sightseeing the South Temple Historic District's churches, houses, and apartment buildings.
4. At this four-way stop, turn right at Virginia St. and cross to the south side of South Temple. For a diversion, The Art Barn is to your south, near the center of Reservoir Park.
5. Proceed west on South Temple's history-lined south side for 1.5 miles.
6. Conclude your walk where you began, at State St. and South Temple.

connecting the walks

Connect with Walk 1, Temple Square, on the northeast corner of South Temple and State St.

Connect with Walk 7, Memory Grove/City Creek Canyon, at State St. and North Temple/Second Ave.

Connect with Walk 13, Lower Avenues, on Canyon Rd. at Third Ave.

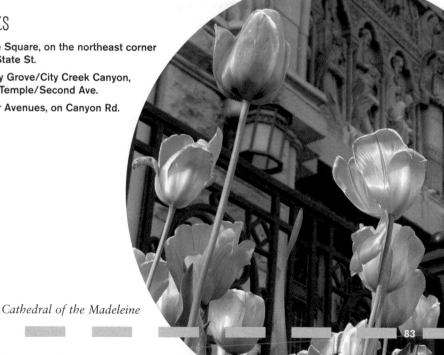

Cathedral of the Madeleine

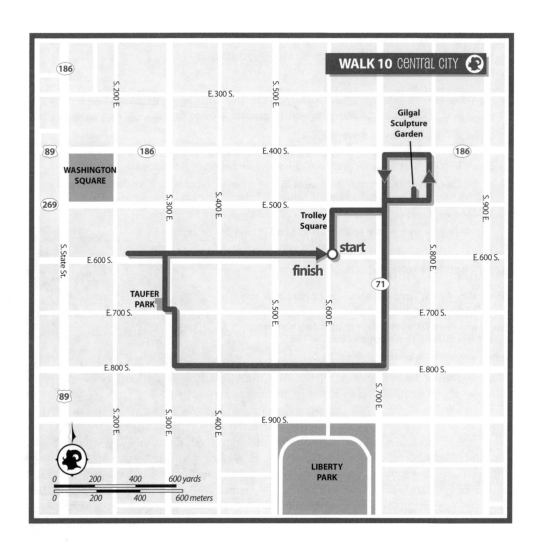

10 Central City: Trolleys Past, Quirky Present

BOUNDARIES: **400 South, 800 East, 800 South, and 200 East**
DISTANCE: **2.5 miles**
DIFFICULTY: **Moderate**
PARKING: **Park free in Trolley Square's terrace lot (the entrance is at about 580 S. 600 East, traveling north); two-hour meters available around Trolley Square, as well as some two-hour free zones nearby.**
PUBLIC TRANSIT: **TRAX light-rail's Trolley Station stop is one block north at 625 E. 400 South on the University Line.**

Let's face it: Utah has a rather conservative reputation. But even in such a setting, and one with a predominant faith to boot, fervor and creativity—entrepreneurial, religious, and artistic—can and do burst forth in surprising ways. Case in point: Salt Lake's Central City Historic District, southeast of downtown. While chockablock with older homes, and certainly not a paragon of wealth, the neighborhood embraces an assortment of innovations and oddities that challenge stereotypes.

Faith-infused Gilgal Garden; a popular corner artesian well; a historic African-American church; boutique businesses; and innovative Trolley Square, a magnetic-trolley and bus barn transformed into a one-of-a-kind mercantile hot spot, give Central City a distinct and quirky character.

Trolley Square is the centerpiece. New stores, additional buildings, and an overall sprucing up have given it yet another recent face-lift. But the heart of the square, and the reasons for its specific "look," go back a full century. The city block itself, along 700 East between 500 and 600 South, was the 10-acre site of Utah's territorial fairs in the 19th century. Once-competing trolley lines merged in 1904 with an electric company, forming Utah Power & Railway Co. (later Utah Light & Traction Co.). Union Pacific Railroad's E. H. Harrison—you may remember his name as the unseen, vengeful magnate out to capture or kill the legendary train robbers in *Butch Cassidy and the Sundance Kid*—stepped into the picture, too. He purchased a controlling interest, as well as the abandoned block, and in 1908, UP&R built the original Trolley Square complex.

This was, for its time, a state-of-the-art "car barn" and machine shop, eventually servicing and storing 144 double-truck trolleys, as Julia Hogan noted in her history booklet, "If Trolley Cars Could Talk: Electric Streetcars and Trolley Square." Mission-style architecture, red brick, arched entryways, and huge skylights gave the mammoth structure its distinctive appearance. Another signature is Trolley Square's almost 100-foot-high, 50,000-gallon water storage tower. Besides helping keep the trolleys clean, the water and the barns' sprinkler system were good insurance against a fire outbreak. Beginning in the early 1930s, however, some trolleys were replaced by the world's first electrified, buslike trolley coaches, which were also stored and serviced here. But the proliferation of automobiles, trucks, and gasoline-powered buses doomed the trolley business. Tracks disappeared from city streets.

In stepped Wallace A. Wright Jr. The developer envisioned new life for the car barns, and they were spared demolition in 1969 when Wright and others, as Trolley Square Associates, converted the site into a lively, antique-filled marketplace, a retro-mall with shops, movie theaters, and restaurants. Paint was sandblasted from the red brick, and trolley relics were rescued and used in the construction, along with wrought iron, woodwork, and glass from several Western mansions and landmarks also on the era's chopping block. In 1973, Trolley Square was registered as a historic site by the State of Utah, and in 1996 it was placed on the National Register of Historic Places. In 1980 it received the Innovative Development Techniques award from the International Council of Shopping Centers.

Today, with a new health-food store and rebuilt parking structures, Trolley Square continues to attract locals and tourists alike. But all around are other interesting neighborhood features, some obvious, others obscure.

- **Begin this walk on the southwest corner of the historic Trolley Square block, at 600 South and 600 East, where metered parking is available on the street, and near the entry to free terrace parking. Proceed north to 500 South and the block's north side.**

- **Turn right to walk east. Cross busy 700 East, a major north-south expressway through much of the Salt Lake Valley. Trolley Corners, a modern complex built to echo Trolley Square, occupies the intersection's southeast corner. Once home to a major movie theater, today Trolley Corners houses a fitness center, restaurants, radio stations, offices, and more recently, Weller Book Works—the modern incarnation of a venerable downtown institution, Sam Weller's Bookstore.**

- Once across 700 East, turn left to cross 500 South, as well, then turn right to walk east on the north side of 500 South. You may encounter delightful aromas wafting hereabouts: A Wonder Bread and Hostess bakery occupies a big slice of this block.

- Continuing east, at 749 E. 500 South, to the left and offset to the north is a path and entry to Gilgal Sculpture Garden. This eccentric but charming little park was once Salt Lake City's "secret garden," tucked away and little-known. The inspiration of Thomas Battersby Child Jr., today Gilgal is fully accessible and landscaped with flowerbeds, stone sculptures, and inscriptions quoting the Bible, the Book of Mormon, and other scriptures. It is well worth a detour. (For more details, see this chapter's Back Story.)

- Exit Gilgal and return to 500 South, turning left to continue walking east. Upon reaching the corner, at 800 East, turn left to walk north. The redbrick Central City Seventh Day Adventist Church is on this corner. Farther along, on the north end of the block, is the chapel of the LDS Church's historic Tenth Ward, founded in 1849. The sandstone and brick meetinghouse, schoolhouse, and store were built in stages between 1873 and 1909. You might also note the Free Speech Zone shop on the east side of 800 East, at 411 S. 800 East. It offers books, posters and other "information for activists, radicals, rebels and rabble rousers," its website declares.

- At the corner, turn left on 400 South to walk west. You are on Salt Lake's "fast-food row." A Chuck-A-Rama buffet restaurant is at midblock, and many other eateries line the street in either direction, from delicatessens and pizzerias to hamburger drive-ins and ice-cream shops. Just beyond the Chuck-A-Rama is a Wonder Bread/Hostess outlet store that provides public access to those wonderful bakery smells permeating the air.

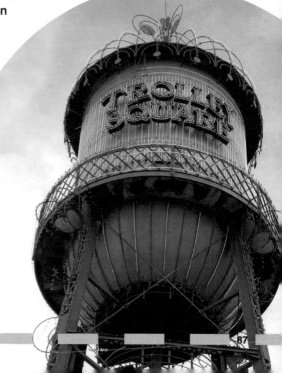

Trolley Square's water storage tower

Back Story

Expect the unexpected at Gilgal, a religious sculpture garden tucked into a lot at 749 E. 500 South in central Salt Lake City. Brimming with iconic statuary—a sphinx-like bust of Mormon prophet Joseph Smith and a Biblical giant broken into a dozen pieces—and engraved scriptures, this is the fantastical creation of Thomas Battersby Child Jr., an architect and stonemason, that makes visible and tangible his deeply held beliefs. The garden is considered by landscape architects and artists to be a visionary art environment.

The dreamscape was laboriously and ingeniously pieced together over the course almost 20 years in the mid-20th century. Child, who also served as LDS bishop of the adjacent Salt Lake Tenth Ward for many years, hoped the garden would inspire visitors to ponder "the unsolved mysteries of life."

"You don't have to agree with me," Child once said of the ideas his garden works espouse. "You may think I am a nut. But I hope I have aroused your thinking and curiosity."

Child began work on the garden in 1945, at age 57, and it subsequently consumed much of his time and money until his death in 1963. For its name,

he chose Gilgal, which means "circle of sacred stones," as mentioned in the Old Testament (Joshua 4:19) and elsewhere.

The intriguing garden includes a dozen original large-scale sculptures, most carved from or constructed using local boulders, with scores of other rocks and flagstones engraved with Biblical and Mormon scriptures, as well as poems and philosophical texts. Biblical figures and references abound, from much-plagued Job to a dreaming King Nebuchadnezzar, as interpreted by Daniel.

Today the flower-graced sculpture garden is maintained by Friends of Gilgal Garden, Utah Master Gardeners, and the Salt Lake City Parks & Public Lands department. The park is open daily 8 a.m.–8 p.m. April–September and 9 a.m.–5 p.m. October–March. It is closed New Year's, Thanksgiving, and Christmas days. Admission is free, though donations are encouraged for continuing maintenance and renovation.

As startling as it is, Gilgal may present too much to soak in during one, or even several, visits. You'll likely leave thinking it is unlike anything you've ever seen before and feeling rewarded for having visited such a place.

- Upon again reaching 700 East, turn left to walk south down the east side of this bustling highway for four blocks, crossing 500 South, 600 South, and 700 South along the way. If you are able to withstand various temptations, you will pass, among others, Litzas Pizza and its sibling Hires Big H drive-in, Ruby River Steakhouse, X-Wife's Place bar, Tucci's Cucina Italiana at Trolley Corners, Elizabeth's Bakery & Tea Shop, and London Market, specializing in British goods. Good luck.

- At 800 South, cross to the southeast corner, turn right at the signal to cross 700 South, and walk west along 800 South. (Large Liberty Park is one block farther south along 700 East). This is a residential area, and quite flat. The colorful little Arts of the World Gallery is one block west.

- On the southwest corner of the 800 South and 500 East junction is brick-lined Eighth South Artesian Well Park. People bring containers large and small (often several) to fill them with the free artesian water spouting here. A sign warns about percolate having been found in the water, "but at levels that studies indicate are not dangerous to public health." That doesn't dissuade too many people, for they park their vehicles curbside and queue up to sip their share. The park is closed 11 p.m.–6 a.m., signs note.

- Continue west another two blocks among the area's compact homes of another era, and turn right at 300 East, crossing 800 South. Stroll north one block to 700 South. After crossing to the street's north side, turn left and cross 300 East. On this intersection's northwest corner is small Taufer Park, a children's playground. On the south side, an old tree has become another object of religious ardor. A makeshift stairway and platform at the tree's base rise about seven feet to a rain-stained bole in which people could discern the figure of a Madonna, the Virgin Mary. A Salt Lake City Parks worker first spotted the icon in May 1997, after lightning struck the tree. Although the image has mostly weathered away, the faithful continue to visit, pasting onto the platform colorful images of Mary and Christ, leaving votive candles, and stopping to pray.

- Return east to 300 East and walk one more block north. Cross to the north side of 600 South, and turn left (west) to walk a few hundred feet to the front of the Trinity African Methodist Episcopal Church at 239 E. 600 South, a National Historic Site. This small brick church, painted a deep red and now engulfed by public education offices and parking lots, dates back more than a century, to 1907. "This congregation has served as a focus of black religious, social, and cultural activity in Utah from territorial days to the present," a historical placard notes.

- Turn around and backtrack east on 600 South, continuing apace for about four blocks, returning to Trolley Square at 600 East. You may notice a sky bridge over 600 South that provides access to the history-laced mall and additional parking on the street's south side. You can either return to your vehicle or explore this quaint retail mecca.

- Trolley Square is certainly worth taking the time at walk's end to shop, window-shop, and dine. The complex boasts several restaurants, from the family-style Old Spaghetti Factory to Rodizio Grill and the Desert Edge Brewery. Shops include Williams-Sonoma and Pottery Barn, and there are gift and specialty shops (clothing, writing paper, linen), an art gallery, a new Whole Foods Market, and much more on two floors and in multiple buildings. To see what Trolley Square originally looked like—car barns, trolley cars, water tower, and all—check out the encased miniature model, near mid-block at the north end of the main building. Railroad hobbyists and kids will love it.

POINTS OF INTEREST (START TO FINISH)

Trolley Square trolleysquare.com, 500 S. 700 East, 801-521-9877

Weller Book Works wellerbookworks.com, 607 Trolley Square, 801-328-2586

Gilgal Sculpture Garden gilgalgarden.org, 749 E. 500 South

Free Speech Zone freespeechzone.wordpress.com, 411 S. 800 East, 801-487-2295

Chuck-A-Rama chuck-a-rama.com, 744 E. 400 South, 801-531-1123

Wonder Bread Bakery outlet hostessbrands.com, 734 E. 400 South, 801-531-6057

Litzas Pizza litzaspizza.com, 716 E. 400 South, 801-359-5352

Hires Big H hiresbigh.com, 425 S. 700 East, 801-364-4582

Ruby River Steakhouse rubyriver.com, 435 S. 700 East, 801-359-3355

X-Wife's Place 465 S. 700 East, 801-532-1954

Tucci's Cucina Italiana tuccis.qwestoffice.net, 515 S. 700 East, 801-533-9111

Elizabeth's Bakery & Tea Shop 439 E. 900 South, 801-433-1170

London Market, londonmarketinc.com, 439 E. 900 South, 801-531-7074

Arts of the World Gallery artsoftheworldgallery.com, 802 S. 600 East, 801-532-8035

Eighth South Artesian Well Park 800 South and 500 East

Taufer Park and **Madonna tree** 700 S. 300 East

Trinity African American Methodist Episcopal Church 239 E. 600 South, 801-531-7374

The Old Spaghetti Factory osf.com, 189 Trolley Square, 801-521-0424

Rodizio Grill rodiziogrill.com, 600 S. 700 East, 801-220-0500

Desert Edge Brewery at The Pub desertedgebrewery.com, Trolley Square, 801-521-8917

Williams-Sonoma williams-sonoma.com, 312 Trolley Square, 801-359-0459

Pottery Barn potterybarn.com, 602 S. 500 East, 801-322-4050

Whole Foods Market wholefoodsmarket.com, 544 S. 700 East, 801-924-9060

route summary

1. Start this walk at Trolley Square, 600 East and 600 South, the block's southwest corner, and walk north to 500 South and the north side of the block.

2. Turn right to walk east, crossing 700 East, then turn left to cross 500 South to the north.

3. Turn right again and proceed east on the north side of 500 South to the Gilgal Sculpture Garden at 749 E. 500 South, if open.

4. Exit Gilgal, returning to 500 South; turn left to walk east, and at the corner of 800 East, turn left and walk north.

5. Turn left at 400 South and proceed west for one block.

6. At 700 East, turn left again and walk south for four blocks.

7. At 800 South, turn right to cross 700 East at the signal and walk west along 800 South for four blocks.

8. At 300 East, turn left to cross 800 South and continue north for one block.

9. After crossing to the north side of 700 South, turn left and cross 300 East to Taufer Park.

10. Return to 300 East and walk one more block north. Cross to the north side of 600 South, then turn left (west) and walk to a church at 239 E. 600 South.

11. Backtrack to 300 East and walk east along 600 South about four blocks. You have returned to Trolley Square, the walk's starting point.

connecting the walks

Connect with Walk 11, Liberty Park, one block south of the southern limits of this walk, at 900 South between 500 East and 700 East.

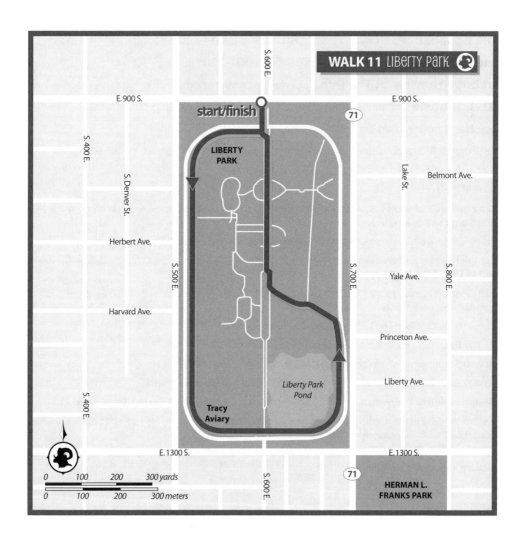

E. 900 S.

S. 600 E.

71

E. 900 S.

start/finish

LIBERTY PARK

S. 400 E.

S. Denver St.

Belmont Ave.

Lake St.

Herbert Ave.

S. 500 E.

S. 700 E.

Yale Ave.

S. 800 E.

Harvard Ave.

Princeton Ave.

Liberty Park Pond

Liberty Ave.

Tracy Aviary

S. 400 E.

E. 1300 S.

S. 600 E.

71

E. 1300 S.

HERMAN L. FRANKS PARK

0   100   200   300 yards
0   100   200   300 meters

11 LiBerTy Park: SaLT Lake CiTy's "CenTraL Park"

BOUNDARIES: 900 South, 1300 South, 500 East, and 700 East
DISTANCE: 1.5 miles
DIFFICULTY: Easy
PARKING: Free inside the park, curbside, and in parking lots
PUBLIC TRANSIT: Utah Transit Authority bus route #9 goes along the north side of Liberty Park, on 900 South. Route 205 travels along 500 East, the park's west side.

With the passing of landscape architect Frederick Law Olmsted in 1903, *The New York Times* praised him and the late Calvert Vaux, with whom Olmsted had designed Manhattan's Central Park, for their vision. "It is to them," the *Times* said, "that we owe the beautiful breathing space" that had become and remains so vital to life in the crowded city. New York City's 843-acre Central Park, which opened to the public in 1859, is credited as the first such urban refuge this side of the Atlantic. It initiated Olmsted's renowned career as a designer of metropolitan landscapes—and became the inspiration for parks throughout the nation.

"Breathing space" is exactly what is offered by Liberty Park, Salt Lake City's little-big homage to Central Park. Opened as a late 19th-century recreational haven in the Olmsted-Vaux tradition, this is a 100-acre refuge of planned forest, grassland, and ponds southeast of the midtown high-rises. It is surrounded by central-city neighborhoods. A variety of recreational activities are available in the park, from soft jogging trails to hard-surfaced paths for biking, skating, and walking, principally along the park's almost 1.5-mile loop. It includes Tracy Aviary, said to be the nation's largest stand-alone aviary, as well as picnic sites, children's playgrounds, tennis courts, and basketball courts. Operating seasonally are a pool and water park, a carousel, and concession stands.

Of course, Liberty Park wasn't always Liberty Park. An 1847 settler, Isaac Chase, was assigned the first five-acre allotment and, with pioneer leader Brigham Young as his partner, operated a flour mill on the site. In 1860, according to a historical marker, Young gave Chase land in Centerville, Utah, in exchange for the house and his interest in the property. The mill and farmland were variously known as Mill Farm, Forest Park, and the Locust Patch. It wasn't until 1881 that Salt Lake City purchased the area from the Young estate to create Liberty Park. The first playgrounds were installed by 1912, and with the automobile age it became a destination for Sunday drives, notes the pictorial history, *Salt Lake City Then and Now*. It remained the community's largest park until Sugar House Park opened in the early 1950s. What is now Hogle Zoo spent 19 years in Liberty Park, from 1911 to 1932, until its animals were moved to new quarters at the mouth of Emigration Canyon. Liberty is "a spacious city park," notes **VisitSaltLake.com,** "with plenty of room for recreation or relaxation," and hosts many community events, from art shows at the Chase Home to come-one, come-all weekly drum circles. Indeed, on July 24 each year the park remains the apex of area Pioneer Day celebrations, the finish line for a marathon and other long-distance races, the site of nighttime fireworks, and brimming with pleasure-seekers.

Note: Vehicles can enter Liberty Park, but access has changed over the years. Today one can park curbside or in small interior lots. However, the north-south artery through the park, 600 East, is now a pedestrian walkway. Also, for traffic control, drivers can no longer cruise the park's oval road in a full, slow loop. Gates at 600 East present a choice for access and parking: east side or west side. For Liberty Park's east side, vehicular entry is via 600 East and 1300 South; you will immediately turn right onto a one-way, counterclockwise half-loop. Ditto for the west-side half-loop, with entry via 600 East and 900 South. For the purposes of this walk, we suggest the latter. Also, dogs are allowed but must be leashed, and you must clean up after them. Alcoholic beverages are not allowed.

- **Begin your walk at 900 South and 600 East, Liberty Park's formal entry. Plaques on tall, flower bowl–topped columns summarize the site's history. Take the sidewalk, just inside the concrete road, for a counterclockwise loop around the park. Across the way, outside of the park, Romney Plaza, a terraced senior citizen living center, is on the northwest corner of 500 East and 900 South. Beans & Brews Coffee House is on the intersection's southwest corner. Houses almost a century-old punctuate 500 East, opposite the park, as does St. John's Lutheran Church.**

- **Looping south, note a side road into the park's center. This offers access to and parking for picnic spots, the Chase Home Museum of Utah Folk Art, and play areas for children (Rotary Play Park's slides, swings, and games) and adults (horseshoes, bocce, and basketball). Just to the south, along the road are the Liberty Park Tennis Center and the park's swimming pool.**

- **Tracy Aviary, which underwent significant expansion and renovation from 2005 to 2011, occupies Liberty Park's southwest acreage and is worth a diversion. There is also a** parking lot to its north. This was the site of the park's early zoo. Tracy Aviary took over the zoo's old quarters in 1938, after local banker Russell Lord Tracy and his wife donated their private bird collection to the city and its children. Today the aviary has about 400 birds, many of them colorful or exotic. They represent 135 species, some rare or endangered, the aviary says. Exhibit areas and pavilions spotlight bald and golden eagles, native Utah birds, South American species, and, most recently, an owl forest. The aviary is open daily, 9 a.m.–5 p.m. Admission is $7 for adults, $6 for children 13 and older and seniors 65 and older, and $5 for children ages 3–12. Children age 2 and under are admitted free. Wheelchairs and wagons are available for rental.

● Outside the aviary, follow the looping walkway south as it curves eastward, to your left. Opposite the park, across 1300 South, should you be in need of refreshment or a meal, are a 7-Eleven convenience store, a popular parkside eatery logically named the Park Café, and other businesses and homes. Some of the aviary's birds are also visible from the public pathway. A little farther away, on the corner of 1300 South and 700 East, is the Adventure Church, a Pentecostal ministry.

● Continue past the wide, two-lane sidewalk at midblock—for now. Until the 1970s this was a road, 600 East, which bisected the park along its north-south axis. Stroll east to the Liberty Park Pond, a haven for geese and ducks and for people who like to toss them a crumb. In 2010 a pipeline ruptured upstream, on Red Butte Creek— coincidentally, during the huge BP oil spill along the Gulf Coast of the United States. Crude oil contaminated the pond's water and threatened wildlife. Almost 200 birds were taken to Hogle Zoo to be cleaned and saved. Work draining, dredging, and refurbishing the pond continued into 2011. As the path loops northward, note the islands in the pond; one has bridge access and a covered terrace. The park's eastern fringe is usually quite noisy, as 700 East is a major traffic corridor.

● Halfway down the park's east side is another sidewalk. Nearby are picnic areas, some with vintage stone pillars, others made of concrete with embedded chess and checker boards. Liberty Park's largest pavilion, Rice Terrace, can seat 200 people. Toward the park's northeast corner are a volleyball court and another small children's playground. However, this side path also offers a fine place to divert west, into the park's interior and the central promenade. Very tall trees line the old 600 East corridor. It is a pleasant walkway in any season, but especially at autumn's peak, when the leaves turn a lovely gold. In the middle of the park are several attractions and points of interest. There is a small, seasonally operated Ferris wheel. In the Seven Canyons Fountain, curves and dips represent canyon-born streams that feed into the Salt Lake Valley's Jordan River. In summer, children can wade in the pool, under adult supervision.

- Just to the west is the park's residential centerpiece, the pioneer-era Isaac Chase home, built from 1853 to 1854. The adobe and stucco residence is one of the city's few remaining houses that date from the 1850s, says one of several historical markers outside. The two-story porch was added sometime in the early 20th century. After 1860, when Brigham Young traded property with Chase, members of the LDS Church leader's family lived in the house. It was later occupied by park employees, by the Daughters of Utah Pioneers, and more recently by the Utah Arts Council. It is currently the Museum of Utah Folk Art, home of the Utah Folk Art Collection, and is open by appointment Monday–Friday, 8 a.m.–5 p.m. To schedule a tour of the exhibits, call Utah Arts & Museums at 801-533-5760.

- Walk a short distance to the south and you come upon Isaac Chase's enterprise, the Chase Mill. It is, according to Tracy Aviary, which now operates the facility, Utah's oldest standing industrial building. Today the restored, adobe-brick structure—with its distinctive gabled roof and big, blocky "B" and "Y" for Brigham Young, its erstwhile owner and co-owner—is used for educational and meeting purposes and can be rented for special events. During the pioneer era, it was a lifesaver. The mill ground grain for the city's settlers from 1852 to 1879. The 1941 edition of *Utah: A Guide to the State,* a Depression-era writers' and history project, says that Chase "transported the millstones and irons across the plains by ox-team. . . . Free flour from this mill saved many lives in a famine winter of the fifties"—meaning the 1850s.

- Return north to follow the tree-lined promenade back to Liberty Park's 900 South entryway. You have returned to the walk's starting point.

POINTS OF INTEREST (START TO FINISH)

Beans & Brews Coffee House beansandbrews.com, 906 S. 500 East, 801-521-5221

Chase Home Museum of Utah Folk Art artsandmuseums.utah.gov, 801-533-5760

Tracy Aviary tracyaviary.org, 589 S. 1300 East, 801-596-8500

7-Eleven 1300 S. 500 East, 801-486-0329

The Park Café theparkcafeslc.com, 604 E. 1300 South, 801-487-1670

route summary

1. Start near Liberty Park's north entrance, at 600 East and 900 South.

2. Proceed west at first, then south, moving counterclockwise around the park's perimeter-loop sidewalk.

3. Consider visiting Tracy Aviary on the park's southwest corner. Or continue on the loop south, then east, to midblock on the park's south side, at 600 East and 1300 South.

4. At Liberty Park's southside midpoint, about 600 East and 1300 South, a wide sidewalk offers a shortcut return to the start, if needed.

5. Otherwise, continue the perimeter walk, east past Liberty Park Pond, and then north.

6. Near midblock on the park's east side is another interior sidewalk, offering easy access to the middle of the park. Turn left here, walking west to Seven Canyons Fountain and Chase Home.

7. Visit historic Chase Mill, south of the residence.

8. Return north to the park's center, and continue north on the central promenade to 600 East and 900 South, the walk's beginning point.

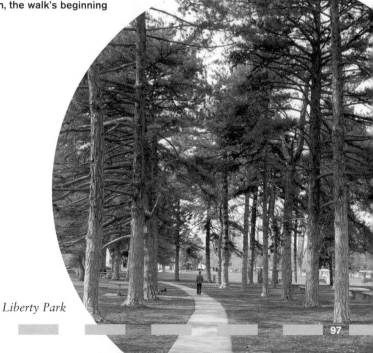

Liberty Park

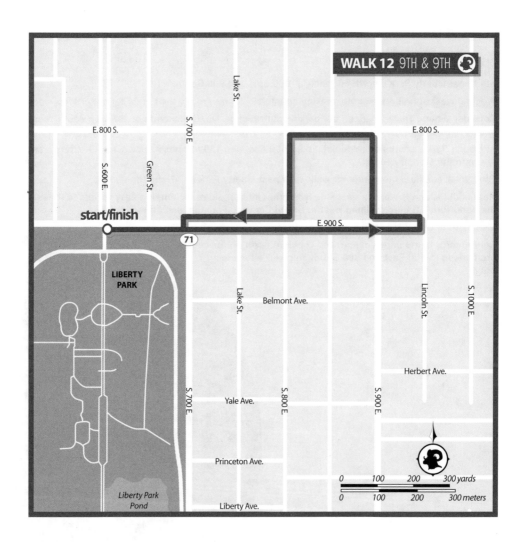

WALK 12 9TH & 9TH

Lake St.

E. 800 S.

S. 700 E.

S. 600 E.

Green St.

start/finish

71

E. 900 S.

E. 800 S.

Lincoln St.

S. 1000 E.

LIBERTY PARK

Lake St.

Belmont Ave.

Herbert Ave.

S. 700 E.

Yale Ave.

S. 800 E.

S. 900 E.

Princeton Ave.

Liberty Park Pond

Liberty Ave.

0   100   200   300 yards

0   100   200   300 meters

12 9TH & 9TH: FUNKY MERCANTILE POCKET

BOUNDARIES: **600 East, 900 South, Lincoln St./945 East, and 800 South**
DISTANCE: **1.2 miles**
DIFFICULTY: **Easy**
PARKING: **Free in Liberty Park; limited street parking**
PUBLIC TRANSIT: **Utah Transit Authority bus route #9 serves 900 South; routes #307 and 320 serve 700 East.**

Before 7-Elevens and strip malls, cities had neighborhood mini–commercial districts, powered by mom-and-pop and family enterprises. Salt Lake City's "9th & 9th"—that's what everyone calls it, centered as it is around the confluence of 900 South and 900 East —is one such enclave that has survived, thrived, and morphed into the 21st century, with a few twists. The more than two dozen eclectic businesses, eateries, and offices that occupy the zone more often than not either have an off-beat countercultural vibe or cater to gentrified tastes.

And *taste* is a key word, as 9th & 9th is a haven for restaurants, delicatessens, and goodie shops serving fare from many lands: Italy, Mexico, Hawaii, and the Middle East, as well as sandwiches and fresh-from-the-farm all-American edibles. Patios and sidewalk seating under awnings and umbrellas are everywhere. Antique buildings house antique wares and consignment goods, as well as funky jewelry stores, barbershops, hair salons, and one of the community's notable, if tattered, film centers, the art-house Tower Theater. Posters and fliers plaster every available wooden power and light pole. In addition, each September, the East Liberty Community Council hosts the food- and music-oriented 9th & 9th Street Festival, promoting neighborhood spirit.

Sidewalks, and even the intersection itself, with a design in its center, underwent a civic upgrade a few years ago, so 9th & 9th sports a spruced-up appearance, with manicured flowerbeds, purple lampposts, and quirky artwork on the four corners. Artist Troy Pillow's slender stainless-steel sculptures depict the nine Muses of Greek mythology. Seven of them have wind-catching kinetic elements that add to their whimsical character. Representing the inspirational daughters of Greek gods Zeus and Mnemosyne, they possess ancient Grecian names like Polyhymnia (the Muse of oratory and hymns, depicted by Pillow with a flowerlike design that seems to have multiple eyes), the free-spirited Thalia (Muse of comedy), and Euterpe (the music

Muse, whose sculpture flutters with colorful paddle-wings). They pay homage as well to Clio, Calliope, Erato, Urania, Melpomene, and Terpsichore. (Remember to enunciate each vowel.)

A saunter to 9th & 9th can begin at pleasant Liberty Park, two blocks to the west, and can even be an extension of a longer walk there, if you have the inclination to browse, dine, or catch a flick in a small mercantile haven with one foot in the past and another in the present.

- Begin this walk in the northeast section of Liberty Park, where there is usually adequate free—and shaded—parking. If driving, enter the park via the southern entrance, at 600 E. 1300 South, following the interior road right (east and then north) to the park's northeastern section to find a parking place. Stroll to the park's north entrance, at 600 E. 900 South, marked by two tall concrete columns topped with flower bowls. Historic plaques on these columns offer an abbreviated history of Liberty Park (the subject of Walk 11).

- At 900 South, turn right to walk east along the street's south side. There is no sidewalk on the park's exterior here, though joggers and walkers have pummeled a distinct path into the grass. Liberty Park's forest of trees adds a bucolic flavor to this bustling city street. Across the way, on the north side, are handsome and generally well-kept residences from the late 19th and early 20th centuries.

- At 700 East, one of the city's heavily traveled traffic corridors, punch the pedestrian-crossing button, watch for vehicles turning from your left, and vigilantly cross to the intersection's southeast corner, to continue walking east along 900 South.

- Continue east, passing tidy homes and crossing little Lake St. (740 East). Some yards have lawns, while others feature planted parking strips and xeriscaped front yards— landscaped mostly with native plants and coverings that conserve water yet offer lovely, often flowering gardens in spring, summer, and into autumn. The walk is ever so slightly uphill, and you will cross a few urban-residential alleys and streets, including quiescent 800 East.

- After traversing midblock Windsor St. (840 East) you arrive at the first businesses in the compact "9th & 9th" shopping district: a boutique; a small Pilates gym; the Thai Garden & Noodle House; a shoe shop; a quaint jewelry store; and Cahoots, a little shop that sells humorous greeting cards, novelties (Salt Lake shot glasses, anyone?), joke gifts, specialty books, jewelry, and more. One of this strip's venerable establishments is Tower Theatre, once a neighborhood movie theater (old photos show that it had crenellated, medieval-looking corner "defenses"). It is now an art-house theater, operated by the Salt Lake Film Society, specializing in foreign flicks, limited-run movies, documentaries, and video and DVD rentals for those who appreciate outside-the-mainstream fare. On the southwest corner of 900 South and 900 East is another veteran, a dry cleaner that has been sprucing up Salt Lake wardrobes "since 1892," a sign advertises.

- At the signaled intersection of 900 South and 900 East pedestrians come across the first of Troy Pillow's metal artworks, depicting the nine Greek Muses. In summer, they rise from luxuriant flowerbeds on each of the four corners. When the signal allows, cross 900 East to the east side. Continue walking east, where you'll find another diverse set of businesses, including several eateries. The corner Dolcetti Gelato shop features "Italian fusion desserts," its signs say. Mazza offers Middle Eastern cuisine. Nearby is Tropical Dreams Hawaiian Creamery, an ice-cream specialty shop based on the Big Island of Hawaii. The Salt Lake shop, according to its website, is the chain's only mainland outlet. A couple of establishments here promote health and inner peace, based on Eastern traditions and New Age metaphysics, with thoughtful (if punlike) names: Centered City Yoga and The Cosmic Spiral. Kitty Kortkamp, at the latter, might sooth your anxious soul with the sounds of the shop's beautiful array of tonal crystal meditation bowls.

- At midblock Lincoln St. (945 East), turn left and gingerly ford 900 South, from south to north, at a pedestrian crosswalk. To be more visible to drivers, grab one of the city's provided orange flags, if there are any to be had. Once you are across the street, turn left to proceed west on 900 South. Businesses here include the 9th South Delicatessen and Great Harvest Bread Co., a bakery and sandwich shop. In summer, a one-tent farmers market sometimes pops up on one lawn, offering local and regional produce.

- Upon again arriving at 900 East (and Troy Pillow's Muses), cross the signaled intersection from its northeast to northwest corner. Restored and trendy businesses here include a children's apparel, book, and gift store on the corner and a substantial bicycle shop. To the west is the Barbacoa Mexican Grill, but turn right after crossing the street to walk north, where you'll note Pago restaurant, advertising "Artisan. Local. Farm Fresh." At midblock is a large Smith's neighborhood grocery store that offers yet more opportunities for food and refreshment.

- At 800 South, turn left to walk west for a block. On the corner of 800 East is Emiliejayne, a consignment shop selling such goods as furniture and home-décor arts and crafts.

- On Emiliejayne's corner, turn left on 800 East to walk south along this quiet street's east side. Salt Lake City is a metropolis of wide streets, a tradition from pioneer times that proved prescient for modern vehicular traffic needs, especially in midtown. However, "Eighth East" is an example of how many of these wide residential neighborhood streets were subsequently divided by grassy medians, in essence miniparks ideal for flag-football games and such.

- At 900 South, where sits the First Christian Reformed Church, turn right to walk past old residences, traversing small outlets like Mendon Court (750 East) and Lake St. (740 East) to hectic 700 East. When the signal allows, cross the thoroughfare to its west side. On the intersection's northwest corner is one of Salt Lake's favorite sweet shops, Cummings Studio Chocolates. Among the specialties, in season, are chocolate-dipped fruit, including strawberries, raspberries, and grapes. Mmm.

- Liberty Park is once again across the way. Turn left to cross 900 South. A diagonal walkway heads southwest toward the park's interior paths, sidewalks, and road—and a return to the section where this walk started.

POINTS OF INTEREST (START TO FINISH)

Thai Garden & Noodle House thaigardennoodle.qwestoffice.net, 868 E. 900 South, 801-355-8899

Cahoots Cards & Gifts 878 E. 900 South, 801-538-0606

Tower Theatre saltlakefilmsociety.org, 876 E. 900 South, 801-321-0310

Dolcetti Gelato dolcettigelato.com, 902 E. 900 South, 801-485-3254

Mazza mazzacafe.com, 912 E. 900 South, 801-521-4572

Tropical Dreams Hawaiian Creamery tropicaldreamsicecream.com, 928 E. 900 South, 801-359-0986

Centered City Yoga centeredcityyoga.com, 918 E. 900 South, 801-521-9642

The Cosmic Spiral thecosmicspiral.com, 920 E. 900 South, 801-509-1043

9th South Delicatessen 931 E. 900 South, 801-517-3663

Great Harvest Bread Co. greatharvest.com, 905 E. 900 South, 801-328-2323

Barbacoa Mexican Grill eatbarbacoa.com, 859 E. 900 South, 801-524-0853

Pago pagoslc.com, 878 S. 900 East, 801-532-0777

Smith's Food and Drug smithsfoodanddrug.com, 876 E. 800 South, 801-355-2801

Emiliejayne 801 S. 800 East, 801-359-3356

Cummings Studio Chocolates 679 E. 900 South, 801-328-4858

route Summary

1. Start in Liberty Park; enter the park via the south entrance at 600 E. 1300 South and (if driving) continue north to park in the northeast section.

2. Stroll north to 900 South, pass the pillared gateway at 600 East, and turn right on the street's south side and walk to 700 East.

3. Cross 700 East and continue walking east to the main 9th & 9th business enclave, crossing 900 East.

4. At Lincoln St. (945 East), turn left to cross to the north side of 900 South.

5. Turn left on the north sidewalk to walk west, again crossing 900 East to the intersection's northwest corner.

6. Turn right, walking north on 900 East to 800 South.

7. Turn left upon reaching 800 South, walking west for one block.

8. At 800 East, turn left onto this residential street and proceed one block.

9. Having returned to 900 South, turn right to walk west to 700 East, crossing this busy street to the intersection's northwest corner.

10. Turn left to cross 900 South, to the northeast corner of Liberty Park. A diagonal sidewalk here leads into the park proper, where this walk began.

Connecting the walks

Connect with Walk 11, Liberty Park, where this walk begins, and to which this walk can be an extension.

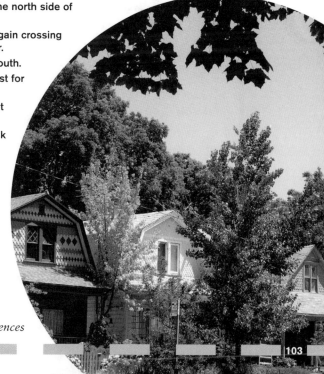

900 South residences

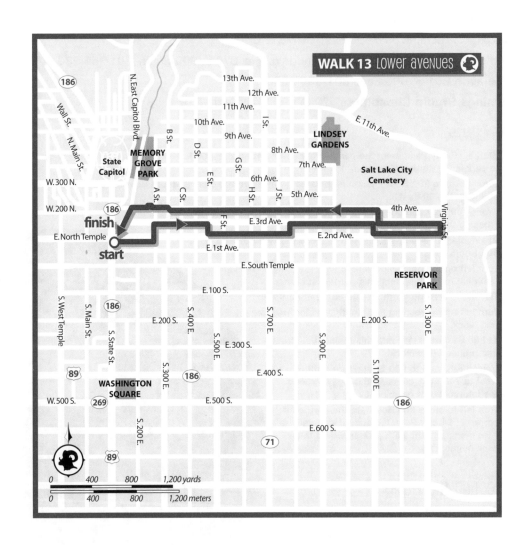

WALK 13 lower avenues

13th Ave.
12th Ave.
11th Ave.
10th Ave.
9th Ave.
8th Ave.
7th Ave.
6th Ave.
5th Ave.
4th Ave.
E. 3rd Ave.
E. 2nd Ave.
E. 1st Ave.
E. North Temple
E. South Temple
E. 100 S.
E. 200 S.
E. 300 S.
E. 400 S.
E. 500 S.
E. 600 S.
E. 200 S.

N. East Capitol Blvd.
Wall St.
N. Main St.
W. 300 N.
W. 200 N.
A St.
B St.
C St.
D St.
E St.
F St.
G St.
H St.
J St.
1 St.

E. 11th Ave.

LINDSEY GARDENS

Salt Lake City Cemetery

State Capitol

MEMORY GROVE PARK

finish

start

Virginia St.

RESERVOIR PARK

S. West Temple
S. Main St.
S. State St.
S. 200 E.
S. 300 E.
S. 400 E.
S. 500 E.
S. 700 E.
S. 900 E.
S. 1100 E.
S. 1300 E.

WASHINGTON SQUARE
W. 500 S.

186
186
186
186
186
186
89
269
89
71

0   400   800   1,200 yards
0   400   800   1,200 meters

13 Lower Avenues: a Pioneering "Suburb"

BOUNDARIES: Canyon Rd., Second Ave., Virginia St., Fourth Ave.
DISTANCE: 5 miles
DIFFICULTY: Moderate
PARKING: Free curbside parking north of South Temple in most of the Avenues area
PUBLIC TRANSIT: Utah Transit Authority bus route #3 runs on Third Ave., from E St. to Virginia St.

"The lower Avenues," on the steepening slopes northeast of downtown Salt Lake City, constitute one of the pioneer community's oldest intact neighborhoods. The streets and blocks were the first to deviate from the valley-floor 10-acre block plan, devised for homes, barns, corrals, gardens, and orchards. Instead, the blocks are only 2.5 acres, and the lots smaller than those below. The people who built their houses here in the Victorian mid-19th century were generally tradesmen, businessmen, and their families, not farmers.

It is, as Karl T. Haglund and Phillip F. Notarianni note in their 1980 book *The Avenues of Salt Lake City,* a unique neighborhood (and one on the National Register of Historic Places) with a delightfully eclectic mix of residential architectural styles. These range from the earliest adobe-brick and simple bungalows to rowhouses and mansions. Mixed in are old-fashioned neighborhood stores with attached houses—the 7-Elevens and Dunkin' Donuts of their era.

However, this area was not originally "The Avenues." Water was scarce. This was "the Dry Bench." And the initial street names differed. At first, all the north-south streets were named after trees: Spruce, Fir, Oak, and Elm were the names of what are today D, E, F, and G streets. The alphabet, at least A through N, had replaced them by 1885. This was also the case for the first east-west streets, originally bearing names like Fruit, Garden, Bluff, and Wall. They became today's Avenues: First Ave., Second Ave., Third Ave., and so on. All of this was codified by the city in 1907, and "The Avenues" had their identity. Trolley cars soon traversed the hillside streets, making living here even easier.

Indeed, the area has the friendly familiarity of neighborhoods portrayed in the movies. Mickey Rooney's Andy Hardy, of the 1930s and '40s, would have felt right at home. But then, so would that goalie-masked teen-murderer Michael Myers, for several of the *Halloween* flicks, set in fictional Haddonfield, Illinois, were actually filmed right here, on the lower Avenues of Salt Lake City.

● If driving, find free curbside parking a half block up Canyon Rd. (a left turn off Second Ave. at 120 East), where there are small median parks and sidewalks bracketing City Creek. Return to and begin the walk at Second Ave. and Canyon Rd. We're suggesting a rather serpentine route at first, turning here and there to savor the old-fashioned flavors of the lower Avenues.

● Go up the street's north side, a rather steep grade for about a block. This was part of Brigham Young's farm a century and a half ago. Today Second Ave. is lined with a diverse cross section of housing. First up on the south, just east of a grassy area adjacent to the corner Brigham Young Memorial Park, is a Victorian-era Queen Anne–style home at 140 East, complete with a bell-shaped roof, stained-glass windows, and iron fencing. Modern high-rise condominiums dominate the north side.

● At the junction of A St. is the campus of today's Madeleine Choir School, until recently the private Rowland Hall–St. Mark's School, itself originally an 1880s girls boarding school. Turn left and go north up A St. a half block on the west side of the street, where a modern LDS meetinghouse stands. Here a marker re-creates part of the thick eight-foot-tall wall that surrounded Young's estate. Originally built in the 1850s "as a protection and make-work project," the wall was "built of cobble stones abounding nearby and laid in lime and sand mortar," the marker notes. Continue north to Third Ave.

● Turn right on Third Ave., walking east on the street's south side. Between D and E Sts. is the Open Classroom Charter School. This has been a school and church site since the 19th century, and for most of the 20th century this was Lowell Elementary School. The neighborhood has kept it alive as a charter school.

● At E St., turn right and stroll south one block to Second Ave. again. A rather Gothic-looking sandstone-and-brick mansion rises on the southwest corner of Second Ave. and E St. As will be typical, large houses mingle with smaller ones, with a sprinkling of retro businesses adding to the mix. At 82 E St., for example, is an irreverent icon: Jack Mormon Coffee Co., a sassy coffeehouse. The aroma of its signature brew wafts through the neighborhood. Art galleries, a preschool, and other enterprises are nearby.

● Cross E St. and walk east along Second Ave.'s north side. As if a counter to the coffeehouse, the handsome (and atypical) LDS 20th Ward meetinghouse, built in 1927 in the Classical Revival style, reposes between F and G Sts. As you continue east on a gradual uphill stroll, the Avenues' miniblocks pass quickly by. At 607 E. Second Ave. is an imposing residence that served as the sheriff's house in movies such as 1988's *Halloween 4.* Note the two lion statues perched on the doorstep.

● Continuing east several more blocks, turn left after crossing K St. and return north to Third Ave. The Wild Rose Bicycle Shop, occupying an old market, and a handy 7-Eleven convenience store across the way add a mercantile lilt to the intersection. One of the reasons for this presence, here and at other points along Third Ave., is that the route, between E and Virginia ("V") Sts., hosted the neighborhood's principal east-west trolley line, beginning in 1890.

● Turn right on Third Ave. and walk east on the south side. At N St., a gas station, the only one remaining in the Avenues proper, continues to serve customers, with an appearance reminiscent of the 1960s. The walk uphill gets a little steeper. The architecture remains varied, with even some simple cinderblock homes thrown in the mix. The intersection at Q St. is highlighted by two large homes on the corners.

● At Q St., cross to the east side and proceed south to Second Ave. once again. Cross to the south side, turn left, and walk east along the avenue. Again, a covey of businesses appear: a laundry, a small office building, and at 1026 E. Second Ave., a gourmet deli. Cucina is open seven days a week, offering espresso, drinks, breakfast, lunch, dinner, and specialty sandwiches, with a friendly, neighborhood ambience. Stray newspapers

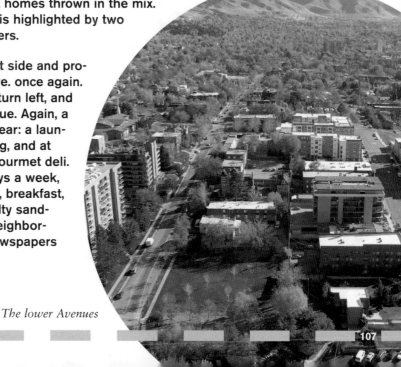

The lower Avenues

Back Story

Salt Lake City's first suburb, "The Avenues," came about in much the same way as urban sprawl happens today: improved services and infrastructure paved the way. In recent decades, where freeways went, water, electricity, and other necessities of suburban life, such as houses, soon followed. Subdivisions were born.

So it was in the 1890s. The Avenues sat on a virtually waterless "dry bench" near downtown, so the first residences clustered near the town's center. But when piped water finally became available from City Creek, the neighborhood grew. The grid of streets expanded north and east, and trolley systems made Avenues life a breeze—before the automobile age sped things up even more.

The city's first trolleys, in 1872, were actually pulled by mules and horses, according to Julia Hogan's history booklet "If Trolley Cars Could Talk." By 1883 the Salt Lake City Railroad Company had 41 cars and 9 miles of track. By the 1890s there were 63 trolley cars and 42 miles of track on the unpaved city streets, Hogan notes. Electrification began in 1889, and route rivalries soon began, with Salt Lake Rapid Transit entering the fray. The companies merged in 1900 as the Consolidated Railway and Power Co., later to merge again with Utah Power Company to form Utah Light and Railway Company.

As early as 1875, the Avenues were key to trolley traffic. The principal line followed South Temple St. to E St., went north up E St. to either First Ave. or Third Ave. (depending on the line and the era) and on to Virginia St. From there, another trolley line took passengers to and from Fort Douglas in the city's eastern heights. Another spur served the upper Avenues, climbing B St. to spurs along Sixth and Ninth Aves. Some routes continued into the 1940s.

The trolley system left a permanent mark on the Avenues, with shops along the lines' routes and slightly wider streets among their legacies. Both the trolleys and the neighborhood were signs of Salt Lake City's transition from a farming village to a thriving center of regional commerce, observed Karl T. Haglund and Philip F. Notarianni in their book, *The Avenues of Salt Lake City*. Growth fostered a diverse, and not strictly Mormon, population of merchants and craftsmen, mining magnates and railroad men, and professionals such as teachers, attorneys, and architects—all of whom called the Avenues home in the late 19th and early 20th centuries and still do so today.

are scattered about. Cozy conversations are shared along the tables near the register and in a long room to the west.

- Continue east on Second Ave. Just past the R St. intersection, glance down to the sidewalk. There for all to see is a sequence of dog tracks embedded in the grainy cement. (Naughty dog!) These undoubtedly date back a century—well exceeding a dozen dog generations. Several fine-looking houses sprinkle these lots, as this was once known as Darlington Place, one of Salt Lake City's first home builder–planned subdivisions. Here Elmer Darling and Frank McGurrin, beginning in the 1890s, bought many lots (whole blocks were not available) upon which they built at least 50 substantial houses for the well-heeled between N and T Sts., and between First and Third Aves.

- At Virginia St.—2.4 miles from the walk's start—turn left and walk north up Virginia one block to Third Ave. (The elegant neighborhood to the east is Federal Heights.) Turn left on Third Ave. and proceed west. On the southwest corner of T St. is The Kura Door Holistic Japanese Spa, another sign of the neighborhood's diversity.

- At Q St., turn right and walk north to Fourth Ave. Turn left on the street's south side and proceed west. Across the way, the Catholic cemetery's southern border is on the north side of the street, as is the Salt Lake City Cemetery adjacent to it farther west. The vintage LDS 27th Ward meetinghouse, constructed in 1902, with a matching cultural hall added in 1927, fills one corner at P St. The Salt Lake Monument Company creates cemetery markers and monuments at N St., appropriately situated across from the main entrance to the city cemetery (the subject of Walk 15). Continue walking west for a straightaway return to this walk's beginning, along a street still rife with the neighborhood's architectural diversity, from simple houses to others with Victorian bay windows and aspirations.

- Across E St., Café Shambala, at 382 E. Fourth Ave., tempts those interested in alternative fare with the spicy aromas of home-cooked Nepalese, Tibetan, and other Himalayan specialties.

- Continue walking west, where between C and B Sts. are 1970s apartments sandwiched between their Victorian-era predecessors. Going steeply but briefly uphill, note the unusual cobblestone Cobbleknoll House on the north side of the street, between A and B Sts. Just beyond A St., Fourth Ave. ends. Descend a few flights of renovated stairs and you are near this walk's beginning. Turn left on Canyon Rd., and within a short distance you are back at your car or starting point.

POINTS OF INTEREST (START TO FINISH)

This Is the Place/Jack Mormon Coffee Co. 82 N. E St., 801-359-2979

Cucina cucinadeli.com, 1026 E. Second Ave., 801-322-3055

The Kura Door Holistic Japanese Spa thekuradoor.com, 1136 E. Third Ave., 801-364-2400

Mt. Calvary Catholic Cemetery mtcalvarycemetery.org, 275 U St., 801-355-2476

Salt Lake City Cemetery slcclassic.com/publicservices/parks/cemetery.htm, 200 N St., 801-596-5020

Café Shambala 328 E. Fourth Ave., 801-364-8558

ROUTE SUMMARY

1. Start at Canyon Rd. and Second Ave. Walk uphill and east on the street's north side.
2. Turn left at A St. and go a half block to a historical marker.
3. Continue north, and at Third Ave. turn right and walk east.
4. At E St., turn right, continuing one block to Second Ave.; turn and walk east on Second Ave.
5. Turn left at K St. and walk north to Third Ave.; turn right on Third Ave. and walk east.
6. On Q St., turn right down to Second Ave. once again; then turn left to proceed east on Second Ave.
7. At Virginia St., turn left and walk up Virginia to Third Ave.; turn left on Third and walk west.
8. At Q St., turn right and walk north to Fourth Ave., following it west to its end.
9. Just beyond A St., descend several flights of stairs to the Canyon Rd. area.
10. Turn left on Canyon a short distance to your car, or the walk's beginning.

CONNECTING THE WALKS

Connect with Walk 7, Memory Grove/City Creek Canyon, at Canyon Rd.

Connect with Walk 9, East South Temple, by walking south to South Temple at any point.

Connect with Walk 14, Upper Avenues, at Fourth Ave. by the Salt Lake City Cemetery, or by walking to Sixth Ave. or Seventh Ave. on the western sections of this route.

Connect with Walk 15, City Cemetery, on Fourth Ave. anywhere between L and U Sts.

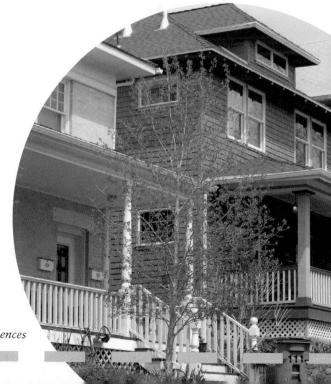

Lower Avenues residences

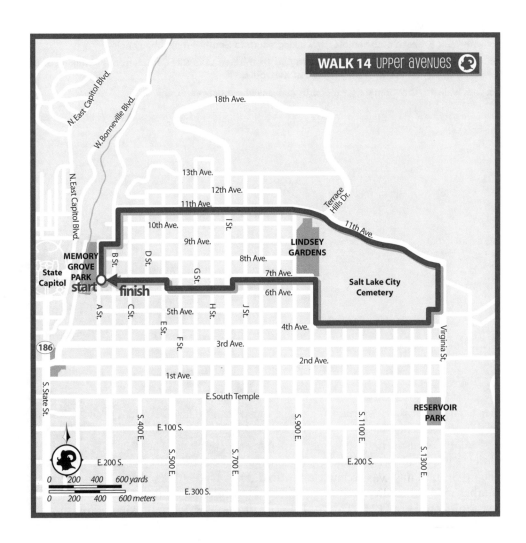

N.East Capitol Blvd.

W.Bonneville Blvd.

N.East Capitol Blvd.

18th Ave.

13th Ave.

12th Ave.

11th Ave.

10th Ave.

9th Ave.

8th Ave.

7th Ave.

6th Ave.

5th Ave.

4th Ave.

3rd Ave.

2nd Ave.

1st Ave.

Terrace Hills Dr.

11th Ave.

LINDSEY GARDENS

Salt Lake City Cemetery

MEMORY GROVE PARK

State Capitol

start

finish

B St.

D St.

I St.

G St.

A St.

C St.

E St.

F St.

H St.

J St.

Virginia St.

186

S. State St.

E. South Temple

RESERVOIR PARK

S. 400 E.

E. 100 S.

S. 500 E.

S. 700 E.

S. 900 E.

S. 1100 E.

E. 200 S.

S. 1300 E.

E. 200 S.

E. 300 S.

0   200   400   600 yards

0   200   400   600 meters

14 upper avenues: roam with a view

BOUNDARIES: A St., Sixth Ave., 11th Ave., Virginia St.
DISTANCE: 4 miles
DIFFICULTY: Moderate
PARKING: Free at curbside along A St.
PUBLIC TRANSIT: Utah Transit Authority bus routes #6 and 11 serve portions of the upper Avenues.

Salt Lake City's "upper Avenues" offer sweeping views of the city and valley below, as well as the Wasatch and Oquirrh Mountains. Snowcapped except in summer, the mountain ranges frame the panorama. Landmarks pop out: the domed Utah State Capitol to the west, downtown's skyline, the University of Utah campus. A vast grid of streets and boulevards rolls into the southern distance. Like the lower Avenues, the high hillside is home to historic residences, diverse architecture, and, on the area's east side, Salt Lake City Cemetery.

Despite a neighborhood retail presence, hospitals actually dominate much of the nonresidential history of the high Avenues. For example, Primary Children's Hospital was located at 320 E. 12th Ave., though its façade dominated 11th Ave. from 1952 to 1990. Today's facility is above the University of Utah campus to the east, and large homes have replaced the original. LDS Hospital, covering multiple blocks around Eighth Ave. and C St., was Intermountain Healthcare's flagship through the 20th century. In 2007 that role was assumed by a new facility in midvalley Murray. Nevertheless, LDS Hospital remains the medical-care heart of the Avenues.

Another early medical linchpin looms at the top of E St., Utah's first Veterans Administration Hospital, which opened in 1932 on 12th Ave. Built at the beginning of the Great Depression, the VA had 104 beds at first, and later expanded to 204 beds. The hospital closed in 1961, and patients were transferred to a new facility on the edge of Fort Douglas on the city's east side. The E St. building was recently renovated, expanded, and converted into condominiums. Yet another medical facility, a modern Shriners Hospital for Children, is on the Avenues' northeastern frontier, at 1275 Fairfax Rd. The orthopedic hospital, which stands on the site of a predecessor, is one of 22 such charities operated by Shriners International, the Masonic fraternal organization.

- Begin this walk at Seventh Ave. and A St., where ample free parking is usually to be found. Walk uphill to the north on A St. Peer down into Memory Grove and City Creek Canyon below, and take in postcard views of the Utah State Capitol and the western horizon. While following the rim of the City Creek abyss, note two different stairways that can safely lead one down into these parks. The distinctive mound-shaped hill to the northeast is Ensign Peak, a prominent summit in Utah pioneer and religious history (and the subject of Walk 8). As A St. dwindles, curve right onto Ninth Ave. and walk east.

- After crossing B St., one of the Avenues' principal north-south arteries, turn left and stride up the street's east side, passing well-kept upscale houses and yards.

- At 11th Ave. turn right, proceeding east. There are no cookie-cutter houses here. Along 11th and above, newer homes of "the Greater Avenues" now cluster in the footprint of the vanished Primary Children's Hospital. The large residences combine both contemporary and early 20th-century flavors and fit in well with older, ivy-covered neighbors. This broad avenue is also a busy route for walkers, joggers, and bicyclists, with marked side lanes dedicated to their pursuits leading to East Bonneville Dr. and the looping one-way road into, and out of, City Creek Canyon.

- At E St., a four-way stop, look north to glimpse Utah's first veteran's hospital. Continue east, where somewhat more modest homes come into view, though the housing theme remains "variety." At F St. a contemporary home is guarded by two lion statues. At 463 11th Ave. East, a cobblestone front-yard terrace adds a pioneer flavor to a cobblestone-pillared home. A Swiss-style chalet rises at 533 11th Ave. East, large pine trees foresting its yard. At I St. towering sycamore trees line the boulevard.

- Continue east. At 830 E. 11th Ave., Salt Lake City Fire Station #4 is on the right. Unexpectedly perhaps, it has a handy vending machine, offering drinks to thirsty joggers and walkers. Across the way, on the hillside above 11th Ave., are an oval running track and a large playground, part of 11th Avenue Park and serving a nearby elementary school. As you continue east, the north side of Salt Lake City Cemetery sprawls along the right (south) side of the road. Some of the upper cemetery wall here was built as a Works Progress Administration project from 1938 to 1941.

- At the T intersection with Terrace Hills Dr., which descends from and rises to the heights to the north, carefully cross left to the north side of 11th Ave. Here the city has created the Greater Avenues Water Conservation Demonstration Garden, a mini-park complete with a seasonal drinking fountain.

- Still on the avenue's north side, but around a curve farther down the road, is a Japanese section of the Salt Lake City Cemetery, complete with a memorial to those who died in World War II. The Garner Funeral Home is just to the east, at 1001 E. 11th Ave.

- Carefully cross 11th Ave. to the street's south side to stroll east along the cemetery wall. This is a favored portion of the pedestrian route used by walkers, joggers, and bikers, in part because of the valley views over the quiet cemetery. Below, a large plat features Salt Lake City's miniature version of Arlington National Cemetery. Uniform bone-white markers, recently restored and brightly complemented with American flags during the Memorial Day weekend, note the graves of casualties and veterans of World Wars I and II. As the cemetery ends, a few houses again line the south side of 11th Ave.

- At Virginia St., 11th Ave. ends. Directly east, across Virginia, is Popperton Park, which represents this area's pioneer name. It includes a continuation of the jogging and walking path, as well as picnic areas, a playground, multipurpose sports fields, and basketball and tennis courts. Just to the park's south is the modern Shriners Hospital for Children.

- Turn right to descend the Avenues hillside southward. Shriners Hospital is across the way, and homes are on the street's west side. South of the medical center and on Virginia

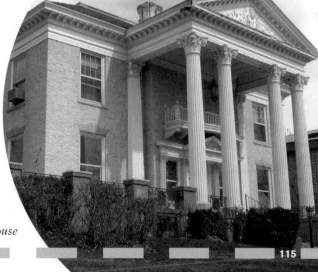

Colonial House

St.'s east side is an opulent yard filled with statuary, including a large figure-infused red heart, statues of painters at work close to the fence with brushes in hand, and a motionless couple, binoculars raised and accompanied by statue-dogs, apparently bird-watching. The mansion was once Utah's governor's residence; today it is the home of a prominent developer and his wife, noted art patrons.

● At Fifth Ave., turn right for one short block, and you are again at the edge of the neighborhood's cluster of cemeteries, in this case Mt. Calvary Catholic Cemetery. Walk south on U St. to Fourth Ave.

● At Fourth Ave., turn right to walk west along the cemeteries' south boundary. You may wish to step onto the boundary road at the entrance to Mt. Calvary for an easier stroll. You will pass by cemetery sections set aside for Catholics (Mt. Calvary) and for Jews (Montefiore and B'Nai Israel cemeteries), as well as the large Salt Lake City Cemetery (the subject of Walk 15).

● At N St., the main cemetery entrance, turn right and walk uphill north to the city park known as Lindsey Gardens, where you will turn left and walk west on Seventh Ave. For a break, consider exploring the small park. An anomaly on the pioneers' "dry bench," a natural spring spouted here. Beginning in 1865, Mark and Birthiah Lindsey began homesteading 160 acres, which they subsequently transformed into the original Lindsey Gardens—one of Utah Territory's first getaways. It included floral beds, picnic areas, playgrounds, bathhouses, and eventually a dance hall. The family sold a few lots for houses, but after Mark Lindsey died in 1878, the family could not retain the land. Some of it was sold for development into small subdivisions. However, community groups petitioned for a park, and in 1921 Lindsey Gardens was reborn on the present site, named in honor of the pioneering couple. Today the park offers tennis courts, restrooms, ball fields, and picnic tables. At the top of a set of stairs on the park's south side along Seventh Ave. is an urn-topped marker noting the efforts of the park's early caretakers, the Flora Culture Garden Club. A twin placard is dedicated to "the women of Utah who served at home and abroad in World War II."

● As you continue west along Seventh Ave., a view of the Utah State Capitol's dome begins to dominate the horizon straight ahead. At busy I St. (the Avenues' "Main St."), turn left and walk down to Sixth Ave. Turn right on Sixth and proceed west. Between F and E Sts. is a Smith's grocery store, by far the largest retail outlet in the Avenues proper—and an excellent stop for refreshments, snacks, and other potential necessities. The level beneath the hillside store houses a Subway sandwich shop, a Utah State Liquor Store, and other businesses.

● If you've paused at the shopping center, return to Sixth Ave. to resume your walk west. At E St., turn right and stride up the steep hill to Seventh Ave. Turn left and walk west. The State Capitol is again in view, and the substantial LDS Hospital complex is on the right. At 259 E. Seventh Ave. is the Colonial House, a striking Classical Revival mansion constructed in the 1890s by mining entrepreneur Gill S. Peyton, though long occupied by the family of investor-philanthropist William H. McIntyre. The colonnaded residence looks as if it could have presided over an antebellum Southern plantation. It has been owned and maintained since 1963 by LDS Hospital, which holds meetings, seminars, and celebrations there.

● Continue walking west on Seventh Ave. to A St., across from the capitol and above Memory Grove. If you drove to this area, you should find your parked vehicle here, where this walk began.

POINTS OF INTEREST (START TO FINISH)

Salt Lake City Cemetery slcclassic.com/publicservices/parks/cemetery.htm, 200 N St., 801-596-5020

Popperton Park 1400 E. Popperton Park Way (360 N.)

Mt. Calvary Catholic Cemetery mtcalvarycemetery.org, 275 U St., 801-355-2476

Lindsey Gardens M St. and 7th Ave.

Smith's Food and Drug 402 Sixth Ave., 801-328-1683

LDS Hospital intermountainhealthcare.org/hospitals/lds/Pages/home.aspx, Eighth Ave. and C St., 801-408-1100

route summary

1. Start at Seventh Ave. and A St.

2. Walk north on A St.

3. As A St. ends, curve right on Ninth Ave. and walk east.

4. Cross B St., and then turn left up B St.

5. At 11th Ave., turn right and walk east.

6. Continue walking east on 11th Ave.

7. At Terrace Hills Dr., carefully cross to the left (north) side of 11th Ave.

8. Continue east a short distance and carefully recross 11th Ave. to the street's south side.

9. Walk east on 11th Ave., past the Salt Lake City Cemetery, to Virginia St.

10. Turn right and walk south down Virginia St. to Fifth Ave.

11. Turn right on Fifth Ave. to U St., then turn left and proceed south.

12. At Fourth Ave., turn right to walk west, along several adjacent cemeteries.

13. Turn right at N St. and walk uphill to Seventh Ave. and Lindsey Gardens.

14. Walk west on Seventh Ave. to I St.

15. Turn left and walk south down I St. to Sixth Ave.

16. At Sixth Ave., turn right and walk west to the Smith's grocery complex.

17. Turn right at E St. and walk one block north to return to Seventh Ave.

18. At Seventh Ave., turn left for a final stretch west to A St. to complete this route.

connecting the walks

Connect with Walk 7, Memory Grove/City Creek Canyon, via either of two hillside stairways descending from A St.

Connect with Walk 13, the Lower Avenues, at Fourth Ave. by the Salt Lake City Cemetery, or by walking to Second or Third Ave. farther west.

Connect with Walk 15, City Cemetery, on 11th Ave., U St., Fourth Ave., or N St. The separate cemetery walk is circumnavigated by this route.

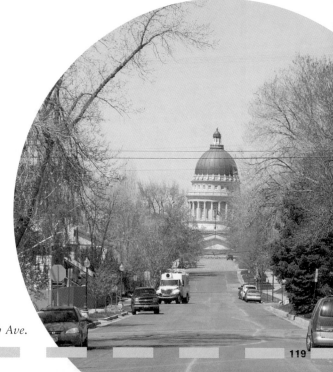

State Capitol, from 7th Ave.

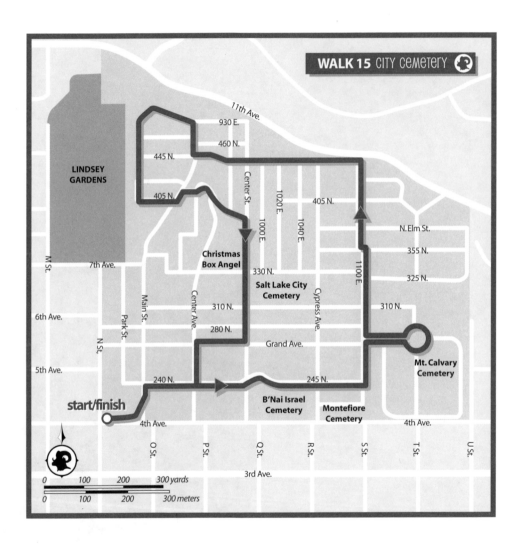

11th Ave.

930 E.

460 N.

445 N.

LINDSEY
GARDENS

405 N.

Center St.

1020 E.

1040 E.

405 N.

N. Elm St.

355 N.

325 N.

7th Ave.

Christmas
Box Angel

330 N.

Salt Lake City
Cemetery

1100 E.

310 N.

M St.

6th Ave.

Park St.

Main St.

Center Ave.

310 N.

280 N.

Grand Ave.

Cypress Ave.

Mt. Calvary
Cemetery

5th Ave.

N St.

240 N.

245 N.

B'Nai Israel
Cemetery

Montefiore
Cemetery

4th Ave.

start/finish

4th Ave.

O St.

P St.

Q St.

R St.

S St.

T St.

U St.

3rd Ave.

0   100   200   300 yards

0   100   200   300 meters

15 CITY Cemetery: Metropolis of the Dead

BOUNDARIES: 11th Ave., U St., Fourth Ave., N St.
DISTANCE: 3 miles
DIFFICULTY: Moderate
PARKING: Park free inside the cemetery, if gates are open, or curbside along Fourth Ave. or N St.
PUBLIC TRANSIT: Utah Transit Authority bus routes #3, 6, 11, and 209 travel near the cemetery.

Founded soon after pioneer settlers arrived in 1847, and draped across 250 rolling hillside acres, Salt Lake City Cemetery is a sprawling metropolis of the dead—though the creators of the tombstone of Thos. A. Tait (1867–90) might beg to differ. "Absent," it says, "Not Dead."

Various publications and websites, such as statistics-oriented **NationMaster.com,** declare this to be the largest city-owned and -operated cemetery in the United States, with more than 116,000 burial sites. Add in the extra acreage of adjacent Mt. Calvary Catholic Cemetery, plus old Jewish and Japanese graveyards, and walkers have an even larger cemetery to stroll. Yes, the U.S. military's Arlington National Cemetery in Virginia, at 624 acres, and a few others, are larger than Salt Lake City Cemetery, but they are run privately or by the federal government.

Though a popular destination on such occasions as Memorial Day and during the Halloween season, a journey through a large cemetery like this can be intriguing at any time, in any season, for it offers a leisurely tour through generations. Salt Lake City Cemetery is sprinkled with markers and monuments paying tribute to prominent families, Mormon leaders, and people of all walks of life, including the occasional scalawag. The epitaphs range from the familiar ("Rest in Peace") to the trite ("Gone Fishin'") to the bizarre ("Victim of the Beast 666"). The stones, and a few rusting cast-iron markers, range from flat slabs to towering obelisks, from Romanesque pillars to Christian crosses, with statuary representing mourning maidens, concerned angels, and Jesus Christ.

The chiseled sentiments are varied. Exemplary mothers and fathers earn high praise. Love never-ending is poetically extolled. And there is positivity from admired orators. For instance, the gravestone of Richard L. Evans, an LDS Church apostle and longtime narrator of the broadcast *Music and the Spoken Word* with the Mormon Tabernacle Choir, bears his familiar farewell, ideal for all occasions—including cemetery rambles: "May peace be with you this day . . . and always."

- Begin this walk at the Salt Lake City Cemetery office, on the grounds' southwest corner, near N St. and Fourth Ave. Receptacles on the south and east walls contain free maps that outline cemetery roads and highlight the burial sites of religious leaders and other notables. (Versions are also inside.) With such maps, you can wander according to your own interests. Note that the cemetery addresses are internal and do not correspond to Salt Lake City's Avenues grid system. Also, the cemetery is built on the side of a hill, so travel north requires an upward trudge. Plan on spending more time here than you might initially expect. There is much to see. The route suggested is far-ranging and counterclockwise. The cemetery is technically open daily from 8 a.m. to dusk.

- From the office's east side and maintenance area, walk up the cemetery's north-south Main St. a short distance, turn right on 240 North and proceed east. Feel free to inspect various intriguing headstones you spot, as time and interest permit.

- At 1100 East, turn left and walk north. After passing 270 North, take the next lane east and turn right into the 19.5-acre Mt. Calvary Catholic Cemetery. A large, dramatic bronze sculpture of the winged archangel Michael hovers near the entry. Crucifixes and angels abound. A roundabout here is actually the cemetery's Holy Cross Plat, a resting place dedicated to the graves of bishops, priests, and nuns. A stone crucifix towers on one side, and at the heart of the circle is an altar memorial to 78 Utah Catholics killed during World War II. In Mt. Calvary's northwest corner are a garden mausoleum, a columbarium for cremated remains, and a lawn crypt.

- After contemplating Mt. Calvary's varied memorials, return west to 1100 East St., the boundary lane, turn right and continue uphill.

- Turn right at 325 North if you would like to take an unusual side tour. Perhaps the strangest headstone inscription in this cemetery complex may be one remembering, as the headstone says "victim of the beast 666." The plot is in the city graveyard's extreme northeast corner, just above the north edge of the Catholic cemetery. The 26th grave in the 14th row states that Lilly E. Gray died on November 14, 1968, at the age of 77. Her tombstone has become legend on the Internet, with more than 2,000 sites now speculating on the "why" behind the devilish reference to the Bible's Book of Revelation. One website's speculation is that the woman's surviving husband blamed police for his wife's death, even though her newspaper obituary states that she died of natural causes in a Salt Lake hospital.

● Return to, or continue north along, 1100 East, moving up the hill. At the top, the road curves west and becomes 445 North St. Follow it, walking west, as you approach row upon row of white headstones standing stoically at attention in the veterans portion of the Salt Lake City Cemetery. This orderly section was recently restored as a service project of several local construction companies. Their names are listed on a marble bench bearing the honest inscription "Freedom Is Not Free." Most of the headstones mark the graves of those who died or served during World Wars I and II, though veterans of other conflicts, before and after, are represented as well. A sliced boulder pays homage to the Gold Star Mothers, those who lost military sons or daughters in wartime.

● Continue west on 445 North until you reach 940 North; then turn right and walk uphill again, angling west on Wasatch Ave. You will pass a north entry to the cemetery, following the lane southwest where it meets Main St. Several late leaders of the LDS Church are buried in this vicinity (as noted on versions of the cemetery map). These include President Spencer W. Kimball and apostles Bruce R. McConkie and Richard L. Evans.

● Proceed south downhill on Main St. At 405 North, turn left and walk east. In the section just to the south are buried two revered, long-serving Mormon leaders, Presidents Gordon B.

City Cemetery

Back Story

Fiction, it seems, can become reality. So Utahn Richard Paul Evans discovered when he wrote the *The Christmas Box* as an expression of love for his two daughters. The story introduced The Christmas Box Angel statue to the world.

In 1993, Evans produced 20 copies of *The Christmas Box* to give as Christmas presents to relatives and friends. Those 20 copies were passed around, hand to hand, over and over. Word spread, and soon bookstores began calling Evan's home to order the self-published book. The short novel was formally published after a bidding war, and became a number one *New York Times* best seller, selling a remarkable eight million copies.

In *The Christmas Box*, a woman mourns the loss of her child, finding solace at the base of the statue of a childlike angel, wings and hands outstretched. Evans says the angel is based on a real statue, though it no longer exists. Grieving parents began seeking out the monument in the Salt Lake City Cemetery. As a result, Evans commissioned just such a statue, and in 1994, the city donated space for it. The popular monument, inscribed with the words "Our Little Angel" on the base, was dedicated on December 6, 1994, corresponding with the date of the child's death in the story. The sculpture was created by Ortho and Jared Fairbanks, a father and son team from Salt Lake City, modeled according to the statue's description in Evans' book.

Hinckley and David O. McKay. Tall stone slabs, very near one another, stand like tabs over their burial sites.

- Follow 405 North east to Hillside Dr., turn north and briefly walk uphill. Soon afterward, turn right on 415 North and enter a small ravine. Continue on the same street as it angles down and southeast to Center St. Along the way you may notice that it is in this ravine where the cemetery stores some headstones or construction equipment, as this is the most obscured area of the graveyard.

- At the junction with Center St., turn right and walk downhill. At about 355 North, on your right to the west, is the Christmas Box Angel of Hope statue. The memorial is to children who have died and is a favored destination of cemetery visitors. The monument

The angel's face is that of Evans' second daughter, Allyson-Danica. Look closely and you can find, on the angel's right wing, the word "hope."

Flowers, sent from around the world, adorn the base of the Salt Lake monument year-round, along with notes and trinkets left by parents in memory of their lost angels. At 7 p.m. on December 6 of each year, a public candlelight healing ceremony is held at the angel statue. Brief remarks are followed by a moment of silence, and a lullaby is sung by a children's choir. Attendees can then place a white flower at the base of the angel statue.

The tradition has spread. There are now dozens of Christmas Box Angel statues, or the "Angel of Hope," at various locations, usually produced and paid for through local donation campaigns. Evans' website says more than 100 are planned around the world.

The Christmas Box was made into a TV movie in 1995, starring Maureen O'Hara, Richard Thomas, and Annette O'Toole. It was the top-rated television movie of the year, won an Emmy, and is rebroadcast regularly, usually at Christmastime.

was inspired by a best-selling book. If you have a cemetery map, it should help you locate this site. (For more about the angel, see this chapter's Back Story.)

- Return east to Center St., turn right and walk down to Grand Ave. (270 North). Turn right on Grand Ave. and walk west. The graves of many pioneers and Mormon leaders can be found near here, including LDS Church Presidents Wilford Woodruff, Joseph F. Smith, and Joseph Fielding Smith (the latter, a father and son). Other notables include John A. Widtsoe and James E. Talmage, both apostles and writers; early pioneer leaders Willard Richards and William Clayton (who wrote "Come, Come Ye Saints"); and notorious gunman-lawman Orrin Porter Rockwell. Again, cemetery maps offer more detailed directions.

- Return to Grand Ave. and walk west to Main St. A left turn on Main will take you south toward the cemetery office and the beginning of this walk.

POINTS OF INTEREST (START TO FINISH)

Salt Lake City Cemetery slcclassic.com/publicservices/parks/cemetery.htm, 200 N St., 801-596-5020

Mt. Calvary Catholic Cemetery mtcalvarycemetery.org, 275 U St., 801-355-2476

ROUTE SUMMARY

1. Start at the Salt Lake City Cemetery office, on the grounds' southwest corner, near N St. and Fourth Ave.
2. Walk north from the office, up Main St. to 240 North, and turn right to walk east.
3. After a slight jog in the road at Center St., remain on 240 North, and at 1100 East, turn left to walk north.
4. After passing 270 North on 1100 East, turn right into the Mt. Calvary Catholic Cemetery.
5. After exploring the Catholic precinct, return to 1100 East, and turn north, continuing up the hill.
6. At the top of the hill, the road curves west and becomes 445 North. Continue walking west.
7. At 940 North turn right to walk uphill, angling west on Wasatch Ave.
8. Follow Wasatch downhill and south.
9. At 405 North, turn left to walk east.
10. Turn left on Hillside Ave. and briefly walk uphill again, turning right on 415 North and entering a small ravine. Stay on the same narrow lane as it angles down and southeast to Center St.
11. At Center St., turn right and walk downhill to the south.
12. At about 355 North on Center St., the Christmas Box Angel is on your right.
13. Continue south on Center St. to Grand Ave. (270 North). Turn right on Grand Ave. and walk west.
14. At Main St., turn left to return south to the cemetery office and the beginning of this walk.

CONNECTING THE WALKS

Connect with Walk 13, the Lower Avenues, on Fourth Ave., the cemetery's southern border.

Connect with Walk 14, the Upper Avenues, on 11th Ave., Fourth Ave., or N St.

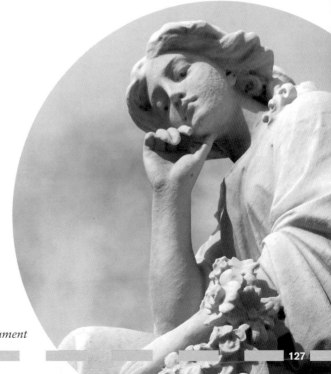

A City Cemetery monument

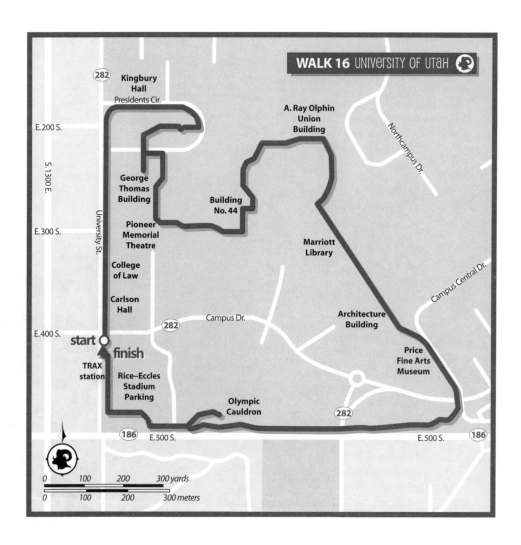

WALK 16 UNIVERSITY OF UTAH

282 Kingbury Hall
Presidents Cir.
E. 200 S.
S. 1300 E.
University St.
George Thomas Building
Building No. 44
A. Ray Olphin Union Building
Northcampus Dr.
Pioneer Memorial Theatre
E. 300 S.
Marriott Library
College of Law
Campus Central Dr.
Carlson Hall
Campus Dr.
E. 400 S.
282
Architecture Building
start
finish
Price Fine Arts Museum
TRAX station
Rice–Eccles Stadium Parking
Olympic Cauldron
282
186
E. 500 S.
E. 500 S.
186

0   100   200   300 yards
0   100   200   300 meters

16 UNIVERSITY OF UTAH: FOR A RED-LETTER DAY

BOUNDARIES: **University St. and Presidents Cir., Campus Center Dr. and the central campus, South Campus Dr. and 500 South**
DISTANCE: **About 2.5 miles**
DIFFICULTY: **Moderate**
PARKING: **Metered street parking of 30 minutes to one hour is available on Presidents Cir. and in small lots; free curbside two-hour parking is available on streets west of campus, but avoid strips with signs noting they are reserved for residents, or you may get a ticket; there are three pay lots on campus.**
PUBLIC TRANSIT: A **TRAX light-rail line connecting with downtown Salt Lake City runs along the south and east sides of campus; Stadium Station is the start for this walk, but there are three additional stations to the University Medical Center. The university has a free shuttle system; for information, visit parking.utah.edu.**

This is a stroll—make that a leisurely procession—through the oldest state university campus west of the Missouri River: the University of Utah. The state's largest institution of higher education, the U of U, or simply the U, is a major research university, with contributions in such areas as medicine (the artificial heart), computer science (graphics and the Internet), and genetics. The school color is crimson. Much of the modern campus was once part of a military camp established during the Civil War, Fort Douglas. So the U, on the hillside bench east of downtown, overlooks the Salt Lake Valley, with outstanding views of the Wasatch and Oquirrh mountain ranges.

Originally named the University of Deseret, when the territory was seeking to be admitted to the union as the State of Deseret, the school was founded in Salt Lake City on February 28, 1850. Deseret is a Book of Mormon word for a honeybee, a symbol of industry to the Mormon pioneers. Classes began in midtown Salt Lake City, about where West High School is today, at 300 West and 250 North. In 1892 its name was changed to the University of Utah, for the territory and, soon thereafter, the state of Utah. The U moved to its current location in 1900 after receiving a few dozen acres of Fort Douglas's western property. Still in use, some campus buildings on Presidents Circle date to that era. By 1940 the U encompassed 143 acres, with about 4,000 students. Today it blankets more than 1,500 acres, enrolls 30,000 students, and has a full-time staff of more than 14,000.

The U was a focal point for the 2002 Winter Olympic Games, hosted by Salt Lake City. Rice-Eccles Stadium was Olympic Stadium. Much of the student housing area was part of the Olympic Village. A visitor center beside the stadium memorializes those heady days.

We can't pass by every one of the U's 300 buildings and sites during our procession—this is simply a slice of what is to be seen on this sprawling, bustling campus. And if you let your feet take you where they will, you can certainly cover whatever serendipitous distance you wish. It is difficult to get lost. Informational signs with maps are posted all around. Maps are available in such locations as the Union Building, the bookstore, and the Park Building, which houses the administration. They are also online at map.utah.edu.

● Begin on the northeast corner of South Campus Dr. (400 South) and University St. (1340 East), walking north. This is just north of the TRAX Stadium Station and is northwest of the Rice-Eccles Stadium parking lot. On the corner is Carlson Hall, built in 1938 as a dormitory and now part of the U's S. J. Quinney College of Law, the principal buildings of which are next. They are followed by the university's Pioneer Memorial Theatre, home of the world-class Pioneer Theatre Company.

● Approach Presidents Cir., which is actually a U-shaped loop. This has been the university's lower-campus core for more than a century. At the head of 200 South, the Circle, as it is known, presents a striking view west into Salt Lake City. Pause at the northwest corner of University St. and the north arm of Presidents Cir. (220 South). To the northwest, on University St., are the Catholic Newman Center for students and an LDS meetinghouse with exterior tile artwork depicting Jesus Christ.

● Turn right along the north sidewalk into Presidents Cir., walking east into a scene that might seem like the cozy collegiate home of movie archaeologist Indiana Jones. The U's oldest buildings are here, and the area comprises the University of Utah Circle historic district. Each building has a historical marker. First up is David P. Gardner Hall, named, as are most of the buildings here, after a former U president. The neoclassical stone structure was built in 1930–31 as the U's Union Building, complete with a cafeteria, a ballroom, a barbershop, and a beauty salon, its placard notes. It served as an Army mess hall during World War II, became the home of the ballet and music departments, and, with the addition of a concert hall, is now the School of Music.

- Next is regal Kingsbury Hall, with four soaring columns, faced in creamy stone in the classical and Egyptian Revival styles. It is named after Joseph T. Kingsbury, the U's president when the university moved to this location. Since 1930 it has been one of the community's important lecture halls and a performing arts center, hosting the likes of Winston Churchill, Eleanor Roosevelt, Robert Frost, and Mikhail Gorbachev. Three thought-provoking slogans are engraved above the front entrance. The center one states, "Learning is ever in the freshness of its youth, even for the old."

- Sandwiched in next, to the north, is a modern building, the T. Benny Bushing Mathematics Student Center. Then come the John W. Widstoe and LeRoy E. Cowles Buildings, both among the Circle's first, built at the turn of the 20th century. The Cowles building served originally as the library, then housed the liberal arts, communications, and mathematics departments.

- As the Circle curves to the right and south, the centerpiece at the top of the looping U is the John R. Park Memorial Building. This colonnaded edifice, which continues to house the university's chief administrators, is named for a pivotal president of the then-young school, John Rockey Park. A formal statue of the educator, boasting a brushy mustache and with a book in hand, stands in a niche beyond great Ionic columns. He was the school's president from 1869 to 1892. If open, consider stepping inside to eye the stately marble interior and five murals, completed in 1940, depicting the advance of culture.

- Farther along the Circle, as it turns west, are the James E. Talmage Building, finished in 1902 as a museum and now a biology center, and the Alfred Emery Building, the then-new

The 2002 Olympics' Hoberman Arch

campus's first building, opened in 1901 to train elementary school teachers. It now houses the Department of Family and Consumer Studies. The final building on the Circle's southwest is the George Thomas Museum of Natural History, a role it recently relinquished. Constructed in 1935 as a library, for 40 years, until early 2011, it housed the Utah Museum of Natural History and its incredible collection of dinosaur skeletons, preserved plants, gemstones, and more. The museum has moved to new quarters, the Rio Tinto Center, and its former building is to be renovated as headquarters for the College of Science.

● Turn around, backtracking a short distance to 1400 East. Turn right at the Alfred Emery Building and walk south. Across the way, to the west, is the William Stewart Anthropology Building (speaking of Indiana Jones). To the left is the Life Sciences Building. After passing beyond the two, turn left and east. A barracks building, used for storage, is to the south. Continue east through a plaza. The modern Biology Building is on your left, and the rounded entry of the Henry Eyring Chemistry Building is on the right.

● Beyond the Eyring Building, and before reaching the Alice Sheets Marriott Center for Dance to the southeast, turn left and proceed north between the brick Biology Building and the Aline Wilmot Skaggs Biology Building, and beneath a skybridge connecting the two. You will enter a more open area of grass and a cluster of trees, many of them planted in honor of university presidents and professors. The U is home to thousands of trees representing the State Arboretum of Utah, and this is a principal grove. Only a few labels remain to tell visitors that they are catching a glimpse of, say, a German ash from the east Balkans.

● Trending east past the Performing Arts Building and the University Campus Store, on your right, shift northeast past a gigantic, sloped granite boulder to the A. Ray Olpin Union Building. Near the south-central entry you might admire *Ute Brave,* a muscular Old West–style statue by renowned Utah sculptor Avard Fairbanks. It is a gift from the post–World War II classes of 1946, 1947, and 1951. A Union Building visit gives you a chance, if you wish, to take a break. Most of the Union Building's food service areas are on this first floor. On the second level are the Union Ballroom and a services desk. There is also a bistro on the fourth floor.

- For continuity's sake, depart the Union Building through the same south-central first-floor entrance, near *Ute Brave.* Walk south toward the U's large, centrally located J. Willard Marriott Library, named for the noted hotelier and philanthropist. The library, which opened in 1968, was recently modernized and seismically strengthened. Walk on the east side of the library and west of Orson Spencer Hall, which houses the College of Humanities, including languages, economics, and politics. You pass through a large plaza with a fountain—and might notice a small sculpture at the corner of one concrete border: a "book" open to pages symbolizing all manner of raised printer's type.

- Continue south (although there is much to tempt you eastward, including the dome-topped Jon Huntsman Center, named for another prominent Utah businessman-philanthropist and home of the U basketball team). As you walk, the Art and Architecture Building will be on your right, and the Business School's C. Roland Christensen Center will be to the left. Directly before you is the Marcia and John Price Building, housing the Utah Museum of Fine Arts. The museum's permanent collection covers a vast span of time, from Egyptian antiquities to contemporary photography, and usually has several exhibits under way at any given time. It has a gift store and a café. There is an entry fee for the museum's exhibit area, which is open Tuesday through Sunday.

- Ready for a sustained walk? Proceed to the museum's east side and resume your southward march along Campus Center Dr., going south. You will intersect with South Campus Dr., a busy junction with a signal, a crosswalk, and TRAX light-rail trains. Cross the boulevard, walking south along 1580 East to noisy, traffic-laden 500 South.

- Turn right at 500 South, heading west—and downhill. Salt Lake City's George E. Wahlen Department of Veterans Affairs Medical Center, named for a World War II Medal of Honor recipient from Utah, is across the busy street, on the south side; farther along is, by comparison, forestlike Mt. Olivet Cemetery. In less than a quarter mile, emblazoned with crimson block-letter U's, is the BCS-buster football team's 46,000-seat Rice-Eccles Stadium—Olympic Stadium during the winter of 2002.

- Alongside the stadium on 500 South is Olympic Cauldron Park, which includes colorful Olympic signage with dynamic images of winter athletes in action, and the metal sculpture known as *Hoberman Arch,* which opened like the iris of a human eye during the downtown medal ceremonies and concerts of Salt Lake City's Winter Olympic Games. The mechanical arch's workings no longer function, but at night, lights play over its gleaming surfaces. Continue beyond the line of athletic images for a view of the towering 2002 Olympic Cauldron, inside a fence. The still-sparkling and jewellike 72-foot tower is faceted with 738 pieces of glass swirling upward toward the sky.

● Continue to the small building nearby on the plaza's west side. The east windows offer a glimpse inside—and into the Olympic Games. This is the park's free visitor center, open Monday–Saturday, 10 a.m.–6 p.m., except holidays—or when Rice-Eccles Stadium is in use. A visit to the center includes a museumlike experience of artwork, historic photographs, and a film. You can also get up-close access to the Olympic Cauldron, now rising beside a seasonal water cascade, with stonework cataloging the names of all the 2002 Winter Games' gold-, silver- and bronze-medal winners.

● Upon leaving the visitor center, walk west through the large Rice-Eccles Stadium parking lot, completing this walk at or near its starting point, at the TRAX Stadium Station and University St.

POINTS OF INTEREST (START TO FINISH)

Kingsbury Hall kingsburyhall.org, 1395 E. Presidents Cir., 801-581-7100

A. Ray Olpin Union Building union.utah.edu, University of Utah, 801-581-7251

Utah Museum of Fine Arts umfa.utah.edu, 410 Campus Center Dr., 801-581-7332

Olympic Cauldron Park stadium.utah.edu, 451 S. 1400 East, 801-581-8849

ROUTE SUMMARY

1. Start at the corner of South Campus Dr. (400 South) and University St. (1340 East).

2. Walk north on University St.

3. At the north end of Presidents Cir., turn right and east to loop the circle, from Gardner Hall to the former Utah Museum of Natural History.

4. Turn around and backtrack east to 1400 East, turn right, and walk south to beyond the Life Sciences Building.

5. Curve east along the sidewalk to a plaza between the Biology Building and the Henry Eyring Building.

6. Take a sharp left and head north, walking between the main Biology Building and the Aline Wilmot Skaggs Biology Building, connected by an overhead bridge.

7. In an arboretum grove beyond the buildings turn east and then northeast, to the A. Ray Olpin Union Building, where you might wish to pause.

8. Upon leaving the Union Building, walk south toward Marriott Library.

9. Continue south, passing between the Art and Architecture Building on your right and the Business School on the left. The Utah Museum of Fine Arts will be before you.

10. Turn left, then immediately right, around the museum to the east-side sidewalk along Campus Central Dr., resuming your way south.

11. Walk to South Campus Dr., cross it at an intersection with a signal and crosswalk, and continue walking southwest along a street marked 1580 East, to busy 500 South.

12. Turn right to walk west down 500 South.

13. Olympic Cauldron Park is on the south side of Rice-Eccles Stadium. Stop by the visitor center if you wish, if it is open.

14. Upon exiting the museum, proceed west through the Rice-Eccles Stadium parking lot to return to the TRAX Stadium Station and University St., the walk's starting point.

The statue, Ute Brave

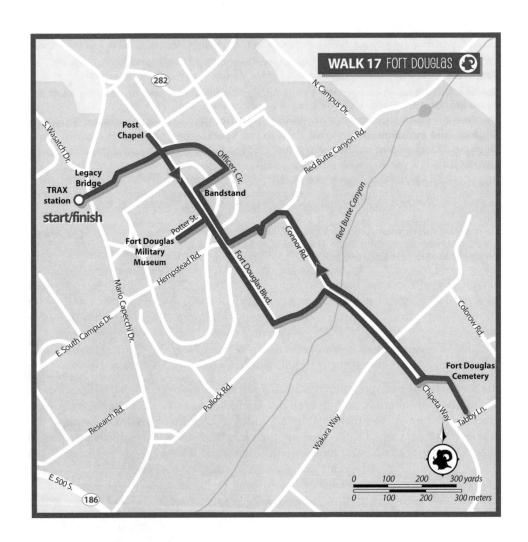

WALK 17 Fort Douglas

282

N. Campus Dr.

S. Waasatch Dr.

Post Chapel

Legacy Bridge

Officers Cir.

Red Butte Canyon Rd.

Red Butte Canyon

TRAX station

start/finish

Bandstand

Potter St.

Fort Douglas Military Museum

Connor Rd.

Hempstead Rd.

Fort Douglas Blvd.

Mario Capecchi Dr.

E. South Campus Dr.

Colorow Rd.

Pollock Rd.

Fort Douglas Cemetery

Research Rd.

Chipeta Way

Wakara Way

Tabby Ln.

E. 500 S.

186

| 0 | 100 | 200 | 300 yards |
| 0 | 100 | 200 | 300 meters |

17 Fort Douglas: a March Through Time

BOUNDARIES: Mario Capecchi Dr., post boundary, Connor Rd./Chipeta Way, Pollock Rd., and Tabby Lane

DISTANCE: 2.7 miles

DIFFICULTY: Moderate

PARKING: Free on streets in western portions of Fort Douglas, especially around Stilwell Parade Ground, and curbside in Research Park to the south; small parking lot west of Fort Douglas Museum and in lots away from student living areas (heed signs about parking restrictions)

PUBLIC TRANSIT: TRAX light-rail system's Fort Douglas Station is northwest of this historic site and at the beginning of this walk; several Utah Transit Authority bus routes and the University of Utah's shuttle system follow Mario Capecchi Dr., on the walk's west side, and Research Park, to the south.

Fort Douglas is a paradox in time. A 19th-century relic, it is part of Salt Lake City, but it was an outside—and outsiders'—community for decades. A discomfiting overseer 150 years ago, even then it provided needed trade and capital for the pioneer settlement. Graced by buildings dating to the 1870s, today it includes and is surrounded by modern buildings and the wizards of high technology, from computer pioneers to genetics miracle-workers. Though built for the purposes of war, it is a peaceful place. As a writer for the *Deseret News,* a Utah newspaper also founded in pioneer times, wrote years ago, "War and bloodshed are just about the last things that come to mind amid the tranquil, parklike setting of Fort Douglas."

And the fort, which once spread across 10,525 hillside acres overlooking Salt Lake City, is no longer a military installation, having been decommissioned in 1991. The University of Utah has benefitted the most. The then-young and growing school was deeded 60 acres in 1894, 32 more in 1906, 61.5 in 1932 . . . you get the idea. With a few exceptions for cemeteries, hospitals, the Forest Service, and the National Guard and Reserve (which still retain a small presence), almost all of that land ultimately went to the U of U. That includes, more recently, the vintage residences of Officers Circle and Stilwell Field, which seem appropriate to a John Ford–directed Western cavalry flick starring John Wayne.

The post was established in contentious times, during the Civil War. Ireland-born Colonel Patrick Edward Connor and his California-Nevada Volunteers were ordered to Utah Territory to guard the overland mail and immigration routes from expected Indian mischief during wartime. The soldiers arrived in October 1862 and set up Camp Douglas, as it was initially called. The name honored the late Illinois Senator Stephen A. Douglas, a proponent of the West who had also been Abraham Lincoln's opponent in the most recent presidential election. But federal distrust of Mormon settlers has also been cited as a reason for the military presence. Placement of the armed camp above the city hasn't discouraged that view. And Fort Douglas, as it was renamed in 1878, thrived. Connor conquered (in one instance, some say, massacred) the area's most restless Indians, kept a watchful eye on the Mormons, and sent out prospecting expeditions, hoping to entice non-Mormons to Utah to harvest the territory's mineral wealth. The California-Nevada Volunteers were succeeded by Army regulars. The fort supported Western cavalry and trained troops during the Spanish-American War and World Wars I and II. Later it served Reserve and National Guard units. In 1970 it became a National Historic Landmark. And in 2002, Fort Douglas was infiltrated by foreigners, as it became part of the Athletes Village during the 2002 Winter Olympic Games and of the university's Fort Douglas Heritage Commons.

As a *Salt Lake Tribune* columnist once observed, Fort Douglas had become a destination for a pleasant and painless stroll through history, with a spacious green parade ground, a bandstand, lovely Victorian brick houses, a historic cemetery, and an enticing museum.

- **Start this walk at the Fort Douglas TRAX station on Mario Capecchi Dr., named for a Nobel Prize–winning U scientist. Nearby is Legacy Bridge, a pedestrian shortcut built just before the 2002 Winter Olympic Games. Unless you prefer a parking spot on the post grounds, step up the western stairway and cross the bridge, which provides easy access to Fort Douglas over the busy six-lane road leading to the University Medical Center to the north. The $5 million, 300-foot George S. Eccles Legacy Bridge features a single-pylon design with cable-stayed suspension. In standard English: The bridge is white with a tall double-post tower, from which are strung weblike cables that support the surprisingly large sky bridge.**

- **Follow the winding path east into Fort Douglas and to the Officers Club, at 150 S. Fort Douglas Blvd. If you haven't arrived via TRAX, bus, or the U proper, and are in a vehicle, park somewhere near the Fort Douglas Museum beside grassy Stilwell Field, named for World War II General Joseph Stilwell, and walk a short distance north along the aforementioned boulevard (a grand name for a two-lane road) to the Officers Club. From the bridge, turn right at the boulevard to the club's street side. The red-sandstone structure was built in 1875 as post headquarters and band barracks. It has had many renovations over the years. In 2001, its front façade was restored, and the building now serves as a conference center.**

- Continue south on Fort Douglas Blvd.'s west side, crossing De Trobriand St. to follow the east perimeter of Stilwell Field, the post's parade ground. Intriguing officers' quarters and barracks line the field, and more are to the east. We will get a closer look at a few of these vintage residences later, but note that Fort Douglas had fallen into disrepair by the late 1990s, when Salt Lake City was named to host the winter Olympics. Many fort residences were refurbished and new housing was built as part of the Athletes Village. After the games, as planned, all became university housing.

- On Stilwell Field's south boundary is Potter St. Cross it and turn right (west) if you would like to visit the free Fort Douglas Museum, which is open Tuesday–Saturday, noon–5 p.m., except federal holidays. Inside are relics from wars fought during the fort's 129 active years. Outside are a statue of Patrick Edward Connor, artillery pieces, two helicopters, four tanks, and other military equipment, all visible to a degree through a fence, even if the museum is closed.

- Return to Fort Douglas Blvd., cross to the street's east side, and continue walking south. The next vintage building to the east is the Post Theater, complete with an old-fashioned ticket booth. Built in 1932, it was a popular escape for military personnel and their families, especially during World War II, a placard notes. The next building is the one-story brick Post Exchange, constructed in 1902. It included a gymnasium. Across the boulevard to the west, behind a high fence, is the still-active headquarters for the 96th Army Reserve.

- Next along Fort Douglas Blvd. are several utilitarian brick structures. First is the brig, a guardhouse built in 1902 to incarcerate up to 40 prisoners. It was more recently converted into a maintenance shop. A bakery follows. First used in 1909, the building

Fort Douglas's Post Chapel

Back Story

The 1863 Battle of Bear River—now more often called the Bear River Massacre—is a little-recalled historic footnote because it occurred during the Civil War, when most Americans were more concerned about terrible battles occurring in the Eastern United States, historian Brigham D. Madsen observes in *Glory Hunter,* his biography of Patrick Edward Connor.

The bloody event was sparked by attacks on miners and immigrants by the Shoshoni Indians of what is today southern Idaho and northern Utah. Many travelers had been killed in Indian raids, and several children kidnapped. Retributory attacks followed against Shoshonis. Pioneers in the Cache Valley, the area around Logan, Utah, also complained of Indian threats, and thefts from farms they had settled. Colonel Patrick Edward Connor and troopers of the California-Nevada Volunteers of Camp Douglas were asked to take action. Connor received judicial approval to do so. The colonel's goal, as Connor says in his own report, was to chastise the Indians—and, Madsen adds, to prove that, as Utah Territory's military commander, he would brook no further raids or killings.

At 6 a.m. on bitter-cold January 29, 1863, after a forced march from Camp Douglas over just a few days and nights, some 200 U.S. infantrymen and cavalry surrounded and attacked an Indian camp on a floodplain along the Bear River near Franklin, Idaho, which at the time was in Washington Territory. The engagement took about four hours. By 10 a.m., at least 250 Shoshoni had been killed—possibly more (one contemporary eyewitness tallied 368)—a great many of them women and children. By contrast, 14 soldiers were killed; many more were wounded or suffered serious frostbite, and several subsequently died. Markers in the Fort Douglas Cemetery list their names. After the battle, the scene descended into disorder. Indian women were raped, historians say. Witnesses reported that soldiers clubbed wounded Indians to death. Connor's brutality and cold indifference to those he considered enemies was one of the military commander's less admirable character traits, Madsen says. Still, the battle was seen as a great victory for Connor and his troops. He was much praised at the time in newspaper reports in California and Utah and was promoted to brigadier general.

was later a motor pool maintenance shop. The street merges with Pollock Rd. and curves left to the east along a parking lot to meet Connor Rd.

- At Connor Rd., turn right and walk south. The route crosses Red Butte Creek and enters Research Park, where former Fort Douglas land is now brimming with modern buildings, with construction crews piecing together ever more. The road's name changes as well, to Chipeta Way. Continuing generally south, you will pass the Williams Companies and Myriad Genetics. Cross through the intersection with Wakara Way. Both Chipeta and Wakara were prominent Ute Indians. Chipeta was the wife and confidant of Ouray, a prominent 19th-century Ute chief. She was sometimes called the queen of the Utes. Wakara, also known as Chief Walker, was a Ute warrior, slave trader, and chief. An 1850s uprising bears his name: the Walker War.

- Cross to the street's east side about a block south, to Fort Douglas Cemetery, with its regimented rows of headstones. *Note:* Rattlesnakes may be in the vicinity during warm months. Signs on the cemetery's perimeter fence warn of the slight danger.

- Enter the graveyard through its northwest corner, marked by a large red history sign with yellow text. There are other entrances, on the south side (Tabby Lane) and east side, where there is a small parking lot, accessible by driving east from this main gate. The four-acre cemetery contains 1,570 burial plots, of which almost 1,400 are filled. The first burial was in 1863. Few are recent, but the entry sign notes the graves' diversity in time and circumstance. "Those officers and men who have died in the service of their country have chosen this sacred and hallowed ground as their final resting place. They represent Civil War, Spanish American War, World War 1, World War 2, the Korean Conflict, and the Vietnam Conflict." A prominent central monument stands in tribute to James Duane Doty, a territorial Utah governor who died in office in 1865. He was a founder of Madison, Wisconsin, had been the governor of Wisconsin Territory in the 1840s, and served in the U.S. House of Representatives. Another tall, carved sandstone marker, topped with a stoic trooper, honors the few Camp Douglas soldiers who died in the Battle of Bear River, just above the Utah-Idaho border. (For more on this battle, see this chapter's Back Story.)

- Explore this evocative graveyard at your leisure. Sadly, many fragile headstones, especially those made of flaking sandstone, are showing substantial weathering, and thus loss of detail. A couple of the most historic plots are on the west side. A monument to Patrick Edward Connor, Camp Douglas's founder in 1862 and later a general, is among these. A tremendous, ragged stone-and-bronze placard bear his portrait, recall his military life, and call him the father of Utah mining. Connor was not always in Utah after commanding Camp Douglas, though he retained an interest in mining ventures. Still, he died in Salt Lake City in December 1891 and is buried here, as are other members of his family. There is another monument to a soldier who perished at Bear River in 1863, and in the southwest corner is a striking 1933 monument, topped by a sad sculpture by Arno A. Steinicke, to German prisoners of war who died at Fort Douglas during World War I.

● Return to old Fort Douglas, first retracing Chipeta Way across Red Butte Creek, but continuing north on Connor St. This area has some of the newest Fort Douglas residential buildings. First is Sage Point, on the left. This housing has three separate buildings, all opened in 2002 for the Olympics as part of the Athletes Village. On the street's right side are seven small older homes or duplexes, built in the 20th century. (Another three such buildings are located a little farther north.)

● At Stover St., turn left toward Fort Douglas Blvd. Turn right (north) upon reaching the boulevard. On the east side, and in the center of the next block, is the Fort Douglas Bandstand. The original grandstand was built in the late 1800s but burned down in 1917, later to be replaced. Until 1940, many Thursday and Sunday evening concerts were held here during the summer months. This replica was built in 2001 as part of the primping before the 2002 Olympics.

● From the bandstand, walk east on the sidewalk to the middle of Officers Circle. Along the crescent before you are 10 nearly identical buildings, used today as honor-student housing at the U. All of the buildings are sandstone duplexes, built from 1874 to 1876 to house Fort Douglas officers and their families. The historic residences were refurbished for the 2002 Olympics. Looming east of Officers Circle is additional midrise housing built for the Olympics, including the Heritage Center. Walk as much of this Victorian circle as you like. Reconnect with Fort Douglas Blvd. on the crescent's north end.

● Turn left to walk north along Fort Douglas Blvd. The post's environmental safety building is on the right. It was originally built in 1904 to serve as bachelor officers housing. Cross the street to the west side to inspect the single-spire Post Chapel, constructed from 1884 to 1886. No longer a chapel per se, this was the longest continuously operating military chapel in the United States Army before it closed in 1991. Renovated in 2001, the chapel is now a nondenominational place of reflection and worship. The chapel's original cross and statue of Christ repose in the Fort Douglas Museum.

● Backtrack a short distance to the southwest, a dry ravine to your right, to connect with the sidewalk used to enter Fort Douglas. Walk west to and across the Legacy Bridge to this tour's starting point.

POINTS OF INTEREST (START TO FINISH)

Fort Douglas Museum fortdouglas.org, 32 Potter St., 801-581-1710

Post Theater universityguesthouse.com, 245 S. Fort Douglas Blvd.; 801-587-1000

Fort Douglas Post Chapel universityguesthouse.com, 120 S. Fort Douglas Blvd., 801-587-1000

ROUTE SUMMARY

1. Start at the Fort Douglas TRAX station on Mario Capecchi Dr. Step up the stairs and cross the Legacy Bridge, walking east.
2. At Fort Douglas Blvd. turn right and walk south.
3. Turn right again on Potter St., beyond Stilwell Field, to visit the Fort Douglas Museum.
4. Return east to Fort Douglas Blvd.
5. Turn south and follow the road until it meets Pollock Rd. and follow it on a short curve east.
6. At Connor Rd., turn right and walk south, across Red Butte Creek, where the street's name changes to Chipeta Way. This is Research Park.
7. After a few blocks, turn left at the entrance to Fort Douglas Cemetery to check out the historic headstones. When you are finished, return to Chipeta Way.
8. Backtrack north on Chipeta Way/Connor Rd. across Red Butte Creek. Remain on Connor Rd.
9. At Stover St., turn left and walk back down to Fort Douglas Blvd.
10. Turn right (north) on Fort Douglas Blvd. Halfway across the distance from Stilwell Field, turn right at the Fort Douglas Bandstand.
11. From the bandstand, walk east on the sidewalk to the middle of Officers Circle.
12. Explore the historic residences on the crescent-shaped Officers Circle, heading to the road's north end.
13. Turn right on Fort Douglas Blvd. and walk north to the Post Chapel, on the west side of the street.
14. Backtrack slightly to the southwest to reconnect with the sidewalk to the Legacy Bridge and the route's starting point.

CONNECTING THE WALKS

Connect with Walk 16, University of Utah, about a half mile west on South Campus Dr.

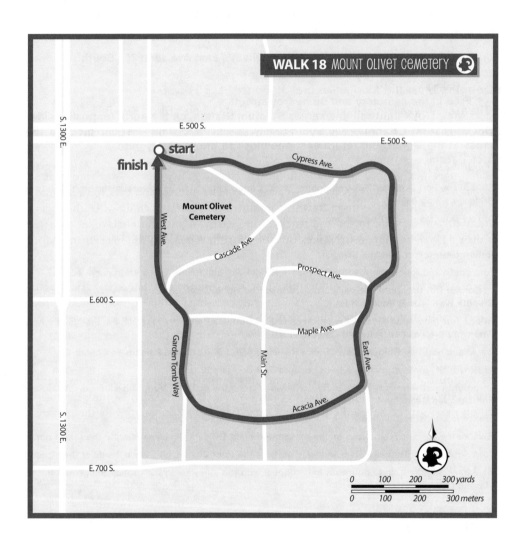

S. 1300 E.

E. 500 S.

E. 500 S.

start

finish

Cypress Ave.

Mount Olivet
Cemetery

West Ave.

Cascade Ave.

Prospect Ave.

E. 600 S.

Maple Ave.

Garden Tomb Way

Main St.

East Ave.

Acacia Ave.

S. 1300 E.

E. 700 S.

0   100   200   300 yards

0   100   200   300 meters

BOUNDARIES: 500 South, University St., Mount Olivet's East Ave., and 700 South
DISTANCE: 1 mile, or as you wish
DIFFICULTY: Easy
PARKING: Free in the cemetery and on nearby streets
PUBLIC TRANSIT: TRAX light-rail line serves Stadium Station, on the north (opposite) side of 500 South. However, to cross 500 South safely, you need to walk west one block to 1300 East, cross at the signal, and return east one block to the cemetery gate.

A historic, parklike gem—a sanctuary unknown even to many locals—lies hidden amid the hustle and bustle of Salt Lake City's busy east side. The intersection of 1300 East and 500 South is a crossroads for commuters and commuter rail, for University of Utah students and workaday folk in cars, and vans and trucks. Yet nearby, a pastoral enclave, popular with urban deer as well as human urbanites out for a stroll, reposes in the maelstrom: Mount Olivet Cemetery.

The U's massive Rice-Eccles Stadium hulks just across the street. The arena roars with people on autumn football weekends. A TRAX light-rail crossing, with a station at the stadium, adds to the metropolitan complexity. They, and six-lane 500 South, require attentiveness from every passerby. By contrast, slip through an obscure gateway into Mount Olivet, at 1342 E. 500 South, and you just might forget all about the hubbub over the fence.

This is an unusual graveyard—said to be the only public cemetery in the United States established by an act of Congress. In the early 1870s, certain residents didn't care for the "Mormon-ness" of the Salt Lake City Cemetery, which was dominated by the territory's dominant religion. Catholics simply created a cemetery of their own, Mt. Calvary, adjacent to the city's graveyard, in what is today the Avenues neighborhood. Jewish congregations and merchants, too, had sections set aside.

Non-Mormons and non-Catholics apparently felt left out. Episcopalians, Presbyterians, Baptists, Methodists, military men, and fraternal societies wanted a final resting place to call their own. They took their concerns to Colonel Patrick Edward Connor of Camp Douglas (later Fort Douglas), the local military post. At first they hoped to get burial space

Back Story

Mount Olivet Cemetery has opted not to create a VIP gravesite map, but if one is familiar with Utah history, a stroll among its intriguing crypts and gravestones offers a roll call of familiar, and often non-Mormon, names. These include some of the state's wealthiest and most influential people: politicians, bankers, and business kings and queens.

Thomas Kearns and David Keith, whose elegant homes are among the grandest on Salt Lake City's elegant South Temple, are buried here. They were partners and mining magnates of the highest order at the turn of the 20th century. Kearns, also a U.S. senator, died from injuries suffered in a traffic accident. Here, too, is Utah Governor George H. Dern, who was Franklin Delano Roosevelt's Secretary of War when he died in office in 1936.

Bankers such as the Walker brothers (several of whom also built mansions on South Temple), Russell Lord Tracy (founder of Tracy Aviary in Liberty Park), and James Collins are buried in Mount Olivet, as are Salt Lake City mayors (among them Ezra Thompson and J. Bracken Lee, who was also a Utah governor) and merchants.

Also interred at Mount Olivet are Elizabeth Dunlap Ferguson Bonnemort, Utah's Sheep Queen, and, somewhere, Her Royal Highness Princess Susanna Egera Bransford Emery Holmes Delitch Engalitcheff, the Silver Queen, whose Park City–generated wealth and lavish parties are legendary. She earned her royal honorific by marrying a Russian prince, who preceded her in death. It is said that her tomb's site is a secret because at the time of her burial there were rumors that she had been buried in a dress made of silver, with silver dollars in her coffin.

in the Camp Douglas Cemetery, but that graveyard was too small to allow nonmilitary burials. So Connor sought permission from the U.S. Congress to donate property on the post's southwest corner for a new cemetery. President Ulysses S. Grant followed through, signing over 88 acres in June 1874. The camp commander and a board of directors, originally consisting of the minister and one layman from each of six Salt Lake–area churches, were to manage the cemetery.

Today the religious concerns of the late 1800s have evaporated. Officials explain that Mount Olivet is a nonprofit cemetery serving people of all denominations and positions in life: Protestants and Eastern Orthodox adherents (Greeks and Slavs), Masons and Moose, African-Americans and Asians—even Catholics and Mormons. It is a peaceful place, with winding lanes and gentle slopes. More than 30,000 souls rest here, with gravestones antique and modern, intriguing family mausoleums, a museum's worth of statuary, and trees of such diversity—almost 90 varieties, according to the Mount Olivet Friends website—that the groves could be considered an arboretum.

Rules more than a century old dictate that dogs are not allowed, nor are unaccompanied children. Horses are not to be left unhitched, or hitched to trees. And as a sign notes, Mount Olivet is open only from 8 a.m. to dusk.

- **Begin the walk within Mount Olivet at the intersection of West and Main Aves. This is just south of the cemetery's main gate on 500 South, near the Tudor-style residence-office. There are informational signs here. Entry is also possible via a west gate at 600 South and University St. (about 1350 East). Parking is available here and there, though the cemetery lanes are narrow. It might be more convenient (and out of the way) to park outside the cemetery's west gate, along residential 600 South, off 1300 East.**

- **Follow Main east a short distance—this is not a large cemetery, so all distances will be relatively short—and keep to the left, where Cypress Ave. branches off, continuing east. (Main Ave. curves to the right, straightening to become the cemetery's north-south axis.) To the left are some of the graveyard's oldest markers, for Civil War veterans in Section A, some bearing the insignia of the Grand Army of the Republic. Other tombstones mark the resting places of those who died at Fort Douglas or those who were lost in or served during the Spanish-American War and World Wars I and II. Over the fence and across 500 South, the U's Rice-Eccles Stadium looms to the north. Surprisingly, because there is a slight rise, or berm, on the grounds' north end, traffic noise is kept to a minimum, undoubtedly a comfort to the herd of deer often seen in this midcity cemetery.**

- **Continue east on Cypress Ave. This is where most of the cemetery's aboveground family crypts are found. The mausoleums vary in architectural style and size. They can house from one to a dozen caskets on the shelves within, notes a guide that is part** of the Mount Olivet Friends website. Masonic monuments are also scattered about the cemetery, along with sections devoted to other fraternal organizations, such as the Elks and the Moose. Along Cypress, for example, is a 1987 Masonic memorial, complete with seating.

● Curve south as Cypress Ave. transforms into East Ave., the cemetery's easternmost lane. The graveyard's oldest graves are in its northeast corner, dating to the mid- to late 1870s, some broken and embedded in the ground.

● As you continue south along East Ave., junctions link to Prospect Ave., Myrtle Ave., and Maple Ave. Feel free to wander the cemetery grounds as your interest, time, and energy permit, for past lives and history are all around. Unlike modern cemeteries where markers are required to be flush with the grass, stonework symbols and statuary abound: maidens and Madonnas, angels and crosses, lambs and doves, tree-trunk replicas and unfinished boulders.

● Walk toward Mount Olivet's southern lanes. Masonic Ave. is the farthest south; beyond is property into which the cemetery can ultimately expand. However, consider turning right (west) onto Acacia Ave., which precedes Masonic. This gives pedestrians a chance to continue strolling along a tree-sheltered lane, with interesting gravesites on either side. Note the variety in headstone sizes, styles, and types. As is true throughout the cemetery, a few markers are metal; most are granite, marble, slate, or sandstone.

● Turn right onto Garden Tomb Way/West Ave. and walk north. There are many flat headstones in this southwestern corner of the cemetery.

● Continue north. At 600 South, the west gate is to your left, if you parked a vehicle there. Cascade Ave. branches off to the right, and this route's starting point is before you. Our contemplative stroll took about 45 minutes. A brisk walk can be much shorter, or you can easily double that if you are interested in the art and history all around in Mount Olivet Cemetery.

POINT OF INTEREST (START TO FINISH)

Mount Olivet Cemetery mountolivetfriends.org, 1342 E. 500 South, 801-582-2552

route summary

1. Start near the main cemetery gate at the intersection of West and Main Aves.

2. Follow Main Ave. east to its junction with Cypress Ave.

3. Keep to the left, angling east on Cypress Ave., the northernmost lane. (Main Ave. curves to the southeast, eventually becoming a north-south road.)

4. Turn right as Cypress Ave. becomes East Ave., walking south.

5. Pass junctions with Prospect Ave., Myrtle Ave., and Maple Ave.—unless you opt to wander and contemplate.

6. Turn right at the intersection with Acacia Ave. and walk west.

7. Turn right on Garden Tomb Way/West Ave. and walk north.

8. At 600 South and before Cascade Ave., the cemetery's west gate is to your left (west), if you parked there. Otherwise, the intersection of West and Main Aves., where this walk began, is a short distance before you.

connecting the walks

Connect with Walk 16, University of Utah, on the north side of 500 South, at the Olympic Cauldron Park, beside Rice-Eccles Stadium. (If walking, it is best to cross this busy highway at the signal at 1300 East, to the west.)

A deer in Mount Olivet Cemetery

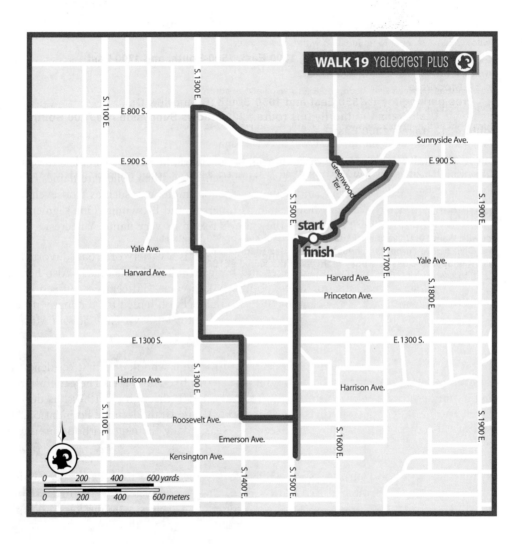

S. 1300 E.

E. 800 S.

S. 1100 E.

Sunnyside Ave.

E. 900 S.

E. 900 S.

Greenwood Ter.

S. 1500 E.

S. 1900 E.

start
finish

Yale Ave.

S. 1700 E.

Yale Ave.

Harvard Ave.

Harvard Ave.

S. 1800 E.

Princeton Ave.

E. 1300 S.

E. 1300 S.

S. 1300 E.

Harrison Ave.

Harrison Ave.

S. 1100 E.

Roosevelt Ave.

Emerson Ave.

S. 1600 E.

S. 1900 E.

Kensington Ave.

S. 1400 E.

S. 1500 E.

0   200   400   600 yards
0   200   400   600 meters

19 Yalecrest PLUS: For the Birds and People Too

BOUNDARIES: **Sunnyside Ave./800 South, 1300 East, 1500 South, and 1700 East**
DISTANCE: **3.5 miles**
DIFFICULTY: **Moderate**
PARKING: **Free parking lot at 1550 East and 1050 South (Bonneview Dr.)**
PUBLIC TRANSIT: **Utah Transit Authority bus route #223 follows Sunnyside Ave./800 South; route #213 travels 1300 East.**

Pleasant residential neighborhoods quilt the heights of Salt Lake City's east side. Among these is an area with an Ivy League air. The streets have been bequeathed collegiate names of the usual suspects, Harvard, Princeton, and Yale; presidential monikers, such as Roosevelt and Harrison; and references to literary lions, such as Emerson and Browning. One segment manages to combine both the Ivy League and the valley's rise in its very name: Yalecrest.

A walk through Yalecrest and onto bordering streets reveals a variety of urban flavors, from lanes dotted with nearly century-old cottages and bungalows to a hidden park. Also here is one of the city's micromercantile hot spots, popularly known as "Fifteenth & Fifteenth." A key neighborhood landmark is the campus of East High School, hailed for the many noted Utahns who are alumni, and recently famous as the stage for Disney's *High School Musical* movie series.

Yalecrest describes most of the neighborhood east of the high school. The first residents settled here in the 1870s, as families took up land to farm five-acre plots. The general area assumed its modern personality in the period from the 1910s through the 1940s, as developers platted and built 22 small subdivisions. According to the Utah Heritage Foundation, the home styles reflect those that soldiers had seen overseas, giving the neighborhood an unparalleled period-architectural variety.

A particular neighborhood surprise is the Miller Bird Refuge and Nature Park, tucked along a half-mile stretch of trail-stitched Red Butte Creek. The pocket was preserved in 1935 by Minnie Miller, a Salt Lake businesswoman, as a home for warblers, woodpeckers, and other birds and as an oasis for residents and visitors interested in a walk through a small, tree-canopied, stream-fed reserve.

- Begin in the Bonneville Glen parking lot off 1500 East and 1050 South (Bonneview Dr.). An LDS meetinghouse with a classic steeple is on the hillock to the northeast. Enter through a gated access. This section is open to walkers and joggers 5 a.m.–10 p.m., a sign notes. According to park rules, pets, bicycles, and smoking are not allowed—though you may see all of those broken during a short walk through the glen and into Miller Park. The path is paved for the first 100 feet, then becomes dirt. Watch for mud puddles following storms.

- Continue walking east. Benches offer sweet spots to rest, meditate, or admire the birds in this forested park. Pass a stone-walled fireplace and curve right then downward to cross the creek. After walking some 300 yards, cross a wooden bridge near a small waterfall. The trail goes uphill and becomes gravel. You will pass several access points and stairways along the way connecting to other sections of Yalecrest. There is a second iron fence access gate, similar to the first one, that leads into Miller Park proper.

- At one-third of a mile out, the trail splits, offering access to either side of Red Butte Creek. The north side seems the most obvious choice. Rushing water drowns urban sounds: You are immersed in nature. A wooden railing borders the path for about 100 feet.

- The trail splits again. Rather than climbing out of the ravine immediately via the left fork, choose the right fork, which descends to a streamside plaza. A plaque details the little park's history. Red Butte Creek, which rises in the hills behind the University of Utah, emerges from a culvert here, from below 900 South and into Miller Park. This is the top of the little oasis that is Miller Park. The walk to this point is just a half mile long.

- Take the stone steps up to 900 South, turn left, and walk west. At the intersection with Greenwood Terrace (1580 East), turn right and walk north one block to Sunnyside Ave., which is the eastern extension of 800 South. Cross to the north side of Sunnyside at the crosswalk to Guardsman Way (also 1580 East), turn left, and walk down Sunnyside Ave.

- Proceeding west you will pass a facility for children with autism on a Guardsman Way corner. The Oquirrh Mountains and portions of the Salt Lake Valley unfold to the west.

You will pass by the new East High School football stadium on the right (north) side; the old high school stadium is on the south side as the road curves.

- At the junction with 1300 East, Sunnyside Ave. becomes 800 South. First Baptist Church, constructed in 1951, occupies the intersection's northeast corner. Cross 1300 East to the west side. A convenience store there offers refreshment and snacks.

- Turn left to walk south on 1300 East. The East High School campus is on the right. The original school opened in 1914. This modern facility is a decade old. Disney's *High School Musical* and its two sequels were filmed in large part at the school from 2006 to 2008.

- Continue walking south down 1300 East, a busy north-south artery. You may notice that the street tops off a valley bench, with steep streets and a sudden drop-off to the west. The reason? Portions of the Wasatch Fault, an ever-present source of earthquakes through much of northern Utah, parallel 1300 South.

- At Yale Ave. (1087 South), turn left to cross 1300 East to the east side. Turn right to walk south, taking time perhaps to note the homes that line the street, most predating World War II.

- At the intersection of 1300 South and 1300 East, cross to the south side and turn left to walk uphill on 1300 South. Cottage- and bungalow-style homes predominate—and many walkers will find it a relief to leave bustling 1300 East behind.

- At 1400 East turn right to resume a southward walk. The street, lined with additional pleasant-looking residences, curves slightly.

Miller Bird Refuge

Back Story

While big-box retail stores and bustling business districts such as Salt Lake City's Trolley Square, The Gateway, and the new City Creek Center downtown claim the lion's share of shopper's attention (and dollars), mercantile nooks such as "Fifteenth & Fifteenth" present a laid-back neighborhood choice for shopping and eating out.

Tucked away on a quiet, tree-lined street, this out-of-the-past yet modern shopping district is one of the city's most enjoyable and varied. Restaurants abound. Here you'll find the white-linen Paris Bistro & Zinc Bar; Caputo's Market & Deli, specializing in Italian cooking ingredients and fresh sandwiches; and an Einstein Bros bagel shop. Across the way is a corner Starbucks. Mazza Middle Eastern cuisine and Fresco Italian Café are temptingly nearby, the latter billed as the city's most romantic restaurant.

Next door to the latter, in a charming, warren-filled cottage, is The King's English Bookshop. Suffice it to say, they don't make them like this anymore. The independent bookshop has tomes of all types scattered about in small, inviting thematic rooms. A popular book-signing venue, it hosts many big-name authors and keeps customers up-to-date with chatty Web alerts from **kingsenglish.com.**

● Turn left (east) at Roosevelt Ave. and walk uphill to 1500 East.

● At 1500 East, turn right to walk south on the west side of the road. After one abbreviated block from Roosevelt Ave. to Emerson Ave., you have reached the quaint retail area of "Fifteenth & Fifteenth," named for the intersection of 1500 South and 1500 East. This is a great place for lunch or a snack, or to pause at a bookshop or an art gallery. On the street's west side are The Paris Bistro, a pet groomery, a clothing store, Caputo's Market & Deli, and Einstein Bros Bagels. On the east you'll find a Starbucks, an art and interior-décor gallery, Mazza Middle Eastern cuisine, Fresco Italian Café, and the King's English Bookshop.

● Cross to the east side of 1500 East and return northward 4.5 blocks to the starting point at 1500 East and 1050 South (Bonneview Dr.).

POINTS OF INTEREST (START TO FINISH)

Miller Bird Refuge and Nature Park utahbirds.org/counties/saltlake/MillerBirdPark.htm, 1500 E. 1050 South

East High School slc.k12.ut.us/schools/high/east.html, 840 S. 1300 East, 801-583-1661

The Paris Bistro theparis.net, 1500 S. 1500 East, 801-486-5585

Caputo's Market & Deli caputosdeli.com, 1516 S. 1500 East, 801-486-6615

15th Street Gallery 15thstreetgallery.com, 1519 S. 1500 East, 801-468-1515

Mazza mazzacafe.com, 1515 S. 1500 East, 801-484-9259

Fresco Italian Café frescoitaliancafe.com, 1513 S. 1500 East, 801-486-1300

King's English Bookshop kingsenglish.com, 1511 S. 1500 East, 801-484-9100

ROUTE SUMMARY

1. Start in the Bonneville Glen parking lot at 1500 East and 1050 South (Bonneview Dr.). On the lot's east side, enter the private but open-to-the-public Bonneville Glen and the Miller Bird Refuge and Nature Park.

2. Walk northeast about a half mile, staying on the north side of Red Butte Creek. At the end of the trail, follow steps up to the sidewalk along 900 South.

3. At 900 South, turn left to walk west. At the intersection of Greenwood Terrace (1580 East), turn right and walk north one block to Sunnyside Ave.

4. Cross to the north side of Sunnyside, turn left, and walk west down Sunnyside, which becomes 800 South.

5. At the junction of 1300 East and 800 South, cross 1300 East to the west side, then turn left to walk south on 1300 East.

6. At Yale Ave. (1087 South), turn left and cross busy 1300 East.

7. Turn right on 1300 East and walk on the street's east side.

8. At the intersection of 1300 South and 1300 East, cross to the southeast corner, turn left, and walk uphill eastward.

9. Turn right on 1400 East to walk south.

10. At Roosevelt Ave., turn left and walk east uphill to 1500 East.

11. At 1500 East, turn right to walk south on the west side of the road to the "Fifteenth & Fifteenth" mini–business district.

12. Turn left to cross to the street's east side, turning left again to walk north.

13. At 1050 South, turn right to return to the walk's starting point.

CONNECTING THE WALKS

Connect with Walk 18, Mount Olivet Cemetery, near 600 South and University St., just north of this walk.

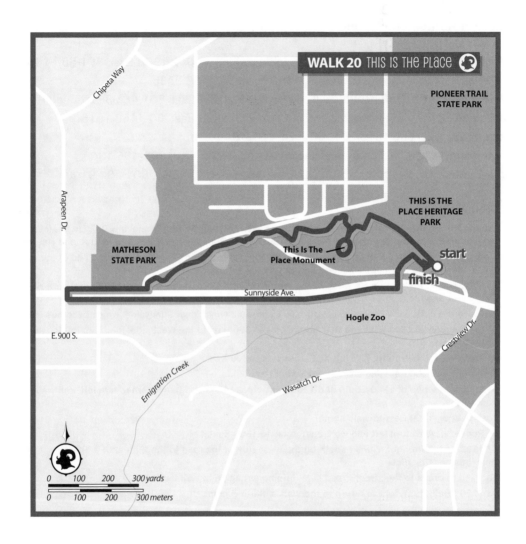

WALK 20 THIS IS THE PLACE

PIONEER TRAIL STATE PARK

Chipeta Way

Arapeen Dr.

THIS IS THE PLACE HERITAGE PARK

MATHESON STATE PARK

This Is The Place Monument

start

finish

Sunnyside Ave.

Hogle Zoo

E. 900 S.

Emigration Creek

Crestview Dr.

Wasatch Dr.

0   100   200   300 yards
0   100   200   300 meters

20 THIS IS THE PLACE: THE "RIGHT PLACE" FOR A SCENIC WALK

BOUNDARIES: This Is the Place Heritage Park, Arapeen Dr., Sunnyside Ave., and mouth of Emigration Canyon
DISTANCE: 2 miles
DIFFICULTY: Moderate
PARKING: Free parking at This Is the Place Heritage Park
PUBLIC TRANSIT: Bus service to This Is the Place and Hogle Zoo is offered 9 times per day (4 morning trips and 5 in the afternoon/early evening) by route #3 of Utah Transit Authority. The bus also offers 3 morning and 4 afternoon runs to the zoo on Saturdays.

Five of the most significant words in the settlement of the American West—"this is the right place"—were uttered here, from a vantage near the mouth of Emigration Canyon. Today, This Is the Place Monument and the encompassing This Is the Place Heritage Park, on Salt Lake City's high east side, commemorate the arrival on July 24, 1847, of Brigham Young, whom colleagues recorded as saying those famous words.

To escape religious persecution, the first Mormon trekkers, beginning in 1846, journeyed 1,300 miles on foot, horseback, wagon, and carriage from Nauvoo, Illinois, to what was for them a promised land. Their route, now the Mormon Pioneer National Historic Trail, took them through what became the states of Iowa, Nebraska, Wyoming, and Utah. According to the National Park Service, roughly 70,000 pioneers took this route before the Transcontinental Railroad made passage easier in 1869. And for many, this was their first good look, after a few high, distant glimpses, at their new home: a sweeping panorama of the broad Salt Lake Valley below, the Great Salt Lake to the northwest, and the Oquirrh and Wasatch Mountains embracing the valley on its west and east sides.

The location makes for a truly scenic walk, and one overflowing with reminders of things past. A massive 60-foot granite shaft, topped with statuary figures of Mormon leaders Brigham Young, Heber C. Kimball, and Wilford Woodruff, dominates the point. Other pioneers, mountain men, Indians, and explorers—including Santa Fe–based Franciscan Fathers Atanasio Dominguez and Silvestre Velez de Escalante, who paused to the south in 1776—are portrayed in bronze around the massive pedestal. The monument, a decade in the making, was designed by Mahonri M. Young, a sculptor grandson of Brigham Young, and dedicated during Utah's centennial pioneer celebration in 1947.

Today, This Is the Place Monument and nearby Statuary Park are the open-to-all areas of This Is the Place Heritage Park, a living-history village of pioneer structures, most of them actual homes and businesses that have been moved here.

But does the iconic monument actually rise where Brigham Young declared the Salt Lake Valley to be "the place"? That's difficult to say, 160-plus years after the fact. The first known marker was belatedly placed in 1917, when Brigham H. Roberts, an LDS Church apostle and scholar, and a troop of Boy Scouts set up a wooden remembrance. Another candidate location is pinpointed by a simple 10-foot-tall, white-concrete obelisk beside a gated service road, amid the oak brush northeast of its more prominent successor. This version was installed on July 25, 1921.

Our walk, including This Is the Place Monument, concentrates on the free stretches along the north and south sides of Sunnyside Ave. This Is the Place Heritage Park is a fascinating and viable walking option as well. The 450-acre village is open daily, year-round, with admission fees based on the day and season. Another option with a fee is just across Sunnyside Ave., the Hogle Zoo.

- Begin this walk from the lower, easternmost parking lot at This Is the Place Heritage Park. If you are driving, entry to the park is on the west, as directional signs indicate. Proceed to the lot below and east of the landmark This Is the Place Monument. Walk west, to and through the main parking lot, to the tall 1947 history icon.

- An optional side trip just to the north, before or after this walk, is to pay the fee to stroll through This Is the Place Heritage Park's village, via the first building you come to, the visitor center. It is a replica of a 19th-century sugar factory. Among the site's homes, streets, fields, outbuildings, and businesses are more than four dozen Old West structures arrayed over the hillside. Some authentic and more than a century old, others replicas, these include the Gardiner cabin, Social Hall, a ZCMI store, Brigham Young's farmhouse, a gristmill, Huntsman Hotel, Deseret Hospital, and the Deseret News Print Shop, as well as Settlers' Pond and a Native American village. Docents are dressed in period costume, food and drink are available, and a replica train can get you off your feet.

● On the main walk, approach the park's centerpiece, This Is the Place Monument. The massive stone pedestal and its crowd of sculptures were dedicated on July 24, 1947, exactly 100 years after Brigham Young's arrival. Delayed by illness, he actually entered the valley a few days after a scouting party that included Orson Pratt and Erastus Snow, who are depicted at the column's base. The monument's east side honors the Donner-Reed party of 1846, which preceded and partially cleared the way for the Mormon pioneers through the rugged Wasatch Mountains, en route to notorious tragedy in the Sierra Nevada Mountains, when the much-delayed wagon train was struck, and stuck, by an early winter storm. Other pieces represent historic figures such as Chief Washakie; mountain men–entrepreneurs William Ashley, Etienne Provost, and Peter Skene Ogden; explorers Benjamin Bonneville and John C. Fremont; and Fathers Pierre-Jean de Smet, Escalante, and Dominguez.

● Continue west downhill to the park's Statuary Walk, a self-guided tour along a sinuous sidewalk. The grassy setting includes numerous statues of many sizes, small to heroic, many of them donated. First up is a tribute to the Willie and Martin handcart companies. Many Mormon pioneers made their way west without oxen, horses, or wagons, pulling their belongings themselves in handcarts. The monument, which includes a handcart replica and a family kneeling in prayer, recalls a tragedy that befell two companies headed to Salt Lake City in 1856. They were caught in an October snowstorm in high central Wyoming. About 210 of 980 pioneers died along the way from exposure, exhaustion, and illness, though many were saved "when rescue parties sent by Brigham Young arrived to help them," a plaque says.

● Among the succeeding monuments is one in tribute to Utah seagulls,

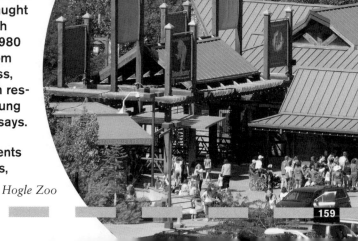

Hogle Zoo

Back Story

Just across Sunnyside Ave., south of This Is the Place Heritage Park, is another Utah treasure: Hogle Zoo, the Intermountain West's largest zoological garden. More than one million people visit each year to see creatures from A to Z—from South America's three-banded armadillo to Zuri, a very popular young zoo-born elephant (who happens to have her own blog: babyzuriblog.com).

Blanketing 42 up-and-down acres near the mouth of Emigration Canyon, Hogle Zoo has a lengthy and colorful history of its own, going back to the early 20th century, when animals were first exhibited at Salt Lake City's Liberty Park. Outgrowing those quarters, the zoo moved to 2600 E. Sunnyside Ave. in 1931.

The oldest building at Hogle Zoo? That would be the zoo's first structure, which still stands as the current Zoo Auditorium. Besides the namesake auditorium, it houses offices and the golden lion tamarin and capuchin monkey exhibits. It is located down from the Hogle Monument, just after the main entry plaza, near the camels. The structure, built in 1931, was originally the home of the zoo's fussy first elephant, Princess Alice, and has been remodeled four times. It has housed lions and tigers over the years and was part of a greenhouse at one time.

Hogle Zoo's miniature railroad has been tooting since 1969. The little train, which can carry 76 passengers at a time, transports about 400,000 passengers each year. The zoo's colorful Conservation Carousel, with painted versions of threatened and endangered animals, swirls almost as many every year: about 320,000 riders.

Many Utahns fondly recall one of Hogle Zoo's most famous longtime residents, and one of the rarest animals in the world: Shasta, a "liger." Shasta's father was an African lion, her mother a tiger. She was born at the zoo on 1948 and died in 1972.

Hogle Zoo seems constantly under construction, as it renovates habitats to better and more naturally accommodate its residents. Recent results have included the Elephant Encounter (Zuri's home), the Asian Highlands, and Madagascar, in the tropical gardens greenhouse.

credited with a miracle for swallowing crickets that were eating precious pioneer crops in June 1848. The birds, a bronzed quotation testifies, "were truly saviors in our behalf, and saved our crops from total ruin." A similar monument is located on Temple

Square in downtown Salt Lake City. The monument Angels Are Near Us, donated by the Sons of the Utah Pioneers, is a large boulder from the original Salt Lake Temple granite quarry. Bronze plaques recognize the participants in the 1997 sesquicentennial reenactment of the original pioneer trek. Other statues honor pioneer settlers and leaders Isaac Barlow and Anson Call.

- A major new monument group down the hill honors the Mormon Battalion, with larger-than-life figures in active poses re-creating farewells and prayers—and one soldier with a gaping hole in his metallic boot, for good reason. During the Mexican-American War of 1846–47, the volunteer company, initially composed of 513 soldiers (along with 33 women and 42 children, one of the artwork's placards notes), marched nearly 2,000 miles. They trudged from present-day Council Bluffs, Iowa, to San Diego, California, "one of the longest infantry marches in U.S. history." The battalion, which fought no battles, built roads and dug wells—and one plaque observes that members were among the first to discover gold in California.

- Continuing west, the dashing Pony Express Monument is next. The statue, based on a 1947 original by Utah sculptor Avard T. Fairbanks, captures a rider and horse springing into action. Riders exited Emigration Canyon and continued into Salt Lake City as part of the Pony Express route between Missouri and California. Although glorified in Western legend, the venture existed for only 18 months from 1860 to 1861—the newly invented telegraph made it obsolete. Just below the monument, placed here in 1998, is a gravel trail that leads to a replica Pony Express station. Built for display during the 2002 Winter Olympic Games in Salt Lake City, the cabin was moved from an Olympics venue to its current location after the competition.

- Pass under the overhead sign and gate marking the entry into This Is the Place Heritage Park, turn right, cross the road, and make your way about 150 feet north to a gravel trail. Turn left to follow the trail west, forking left again soon after, heading toward Sunnyside Ave. The path is part of the Scott M. Matheson Nature Preserve and Governors Grove Trail, honoring Utah's 12th governor. (Another section of the trail loops around a field.)

- Leave the trail as it connects with Sunnyside Ave. Turn right and carefully walk down the north side of the street, a short roadside trail and lawn lacking a sidewalk, heading west. A U.S. Postal Service office is here, on the northeast corner of the intersection of Sunnyside Ave. and Arapeen Dr.

● At the intersection signal, turn left to cross to the south side of Sunnyside Ave., then turn left again to walk east up the inclined sidewalk toward the mouth of Emigration Canyon. Along the way are some impressive modern homes, and, after about a half mile, the northern fence line of Hogle Zoo. The first zoo building is the animal hospital . . . and beyond, some rather pungent zoological odors. (The elephant quarters are nearby.)

● Just under a mile up Sunnyside, along the side of the zoo's parking lot, is a button-operated signal for a pedestrian crossing. Be aware: Pushing the button to cross does not create a red light for cars along Sunnyside, but it does flash a yellow caution light. After looking both ways to be sure vehicles are indeed stopping, cross north toward the This Is the Place Heritage Park parking lot. Walk up a set of stairs, and you have returned to this walk's starting point.

● Here's another option: The small 1921 This Is the Place Monument, which may more closely mark the spot where Brigham Young declared "This is the right place," is just up the short paved road northeast of the lower, eastern parking lot where this walk began. Pass by the arm of the single-post gate preventing motorized entry. Walk about 120 yards around the corner and look for the bright-white obelisk on the right (east) side of the road. A plaque on the monument, refurbished and rededicated in 1997, declares the spot to be the most definitive location of Brigham Young's declaration. This is based upon newspaper stories relating the recollections of W. W. Riter, who was "a lad of 9," a placard says, when he arrived with his parents and often visited the site with pioneer leader Wilford Woodruff, and of historian and theologian Brigham H. Roberts, who had placed a wooden marker with a troop of Scouts a few years before. The round-trip distance of this side trip is about 0.2 mile from the parking lot, though it is slightly uphill to the white obelisk.

POINTS OF INTEREST (start to finish)

This Is the Place Heritage Park thisistheplace.org, 2601 E. Sunnyside Ave., 801-582-1847

Hogle Zoo hoglezoo.org, 2600 E. Sunnyside Ave., 801-582-1631

route summary

1. Start from the easternmost lower-level parking lot at This Is the Place Heritage Park. Walk west, through the main parking lot, to This Is the Place Monument.

2. An optional side trip, before or after this walk, is to pay the fee in the visitor center near the parking lot, and tour the park's pioneer village to the north.

3. Inspect This Is the Place Monument.

4. Continue west to the park's Statuary Walk, following the curving sidewalk among the statues and monuments.

5. Cross under the gateway marking the entrance to This Is the Place Heritage Park and turn right to cross the road.

6. Cross a short patch of grass and dirt about 150 feet to the north to connect with a gravel trail that is part of the Scott M. Matheson Preserve and Governors Grove.

7. Turn left and follow the trail west, forking left again soon after, toward Sunnyside Ave.

8. Leave the formal trail at Sunnyside Ave. Turn right and carefully walk down the north side of the road or along a short dirt-and-grass trail or grass, heading west.

9. At the signal intersection of Sunnyside Ave. and Arapeen Dr., turn left to cross to the south side of Sunnyside Ave.

10. On the avenue's south side, turn left again to walk east uphill, along a sidewalk, toward the mouth of Emigration Canyon, for just under a mile.

11. Pass Hogle Zoo's northern fences, to a lighted pedestrian crosswalk with an operational button, outside the zoo parking lot. The signal is a flashing yellow light for both crossing pedestrians and oncoming traffic.

12. Cross Sunnyside Ave. north, looking carefully both ways to be sure vehicles are stopping.

13. On the north side of Sunnyside Ave., walk up a set of stairs, and you have returned to the lower parking lot of This Is the Place Heritage Park, your starting point.

14. A short 0.2-mile option nearby is to walk to the parking lot's northeast corner to a short, gated service road that offers access to a small 1921 This Is the Place Monument, then to return to the parking lot.

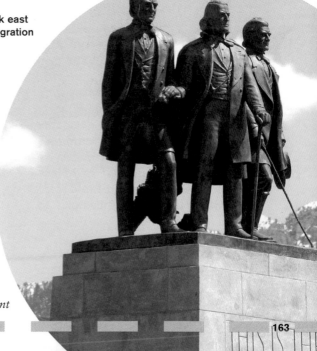

The top of This Is the Place Monument

163

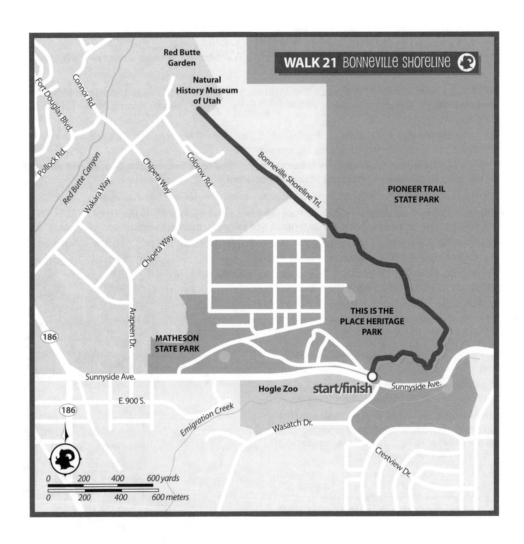

Red Butte
Garden

Natural
History Museum
of Utah

Fort Douglas Blvd.

Connor Rd.

Pollock Rd.

Red Butte Canyon

Wakara Way

Chipeta Way

Colorow Rd.

Bonneville Shoreline Trl.

PIONEER TRAIL
STATE PARK

Chipeta Way

Arapeen Dr.

186

THIS IS THE
PLACE HERITAGE
PARK

MATHESON
STATE PARK

Sunnyside Ave.

186

E. 900 S.

Hogle Zoo

Emigration Creek

start/finish

Sunnyside Ave.

Wasatch Dr.

Crestview Dr.

0   200   400   600 yards

0   200   400   600 meters

21 BONNEVILLE SHORELINE: A CITY LAPPING AT YOUR FEET

BOUNDARIES: Sunnyside Ave., Wasatch Mountains, Wakara Way; This Is the Place Heritage Park and Red Butte Garden
DISTANCE: 3.6 miles
DIFFICULTY: Strenuous
PARKING: Free in trailhead lot or along Sunnyside Ave.
PUBLIC TRANSIT: Utah Transit Authority bus route #228 serves Sunnyside Ave. in the summer only; route #3 serves Research Park, about a mile below the trailhead.

Imagine the Salt Lake Valley under 1,000 feet of water. Envision most of western Utah submerged as well, not from a flood, but from a sprawling, ancient inland sea we today call Lake Bonneville. The mountain ranges to your west would be long islands. Today's Bonneville Shoreline Trail would be along, or under, the beaches and fringes of that vast, prehistoric lake. Nowadays, instead of water, Salt Lake City and its suburbs lap at your feet.

Lake Bonneville filled these valleys during the last Ice Age, from 7,000 to 28,000 years ago. The lake gradually vanished during a long decline. A natural dam broke. The cooler, wetter climate changed to a warmer, dryer one. The Great Salt Lake is its largest remnant, though Bonneville left behind other evidence, from Utah's desert salt flats to various mountainside terraces, which highlight its shoreline at various levels. The highest ancient beach is at 5,200 feet above sea level—the Bonneville level, from about 16,800 to 18,000 years ago.

The Bonneville Shoreline Trail, with its fine views of downtown Salt Lake City, is one of Utah's longest, with a potential length of 280 miles, stretching from the Idaho border to Nephi. The trail's concept emerged in 1990, during a controversy involving possible restrictions on the heavily used hiking, jogging, and biking foothill path between Emigration Canyon on the south and Dry Canyon on the north. This Is the Place State Park, as it was called at the time, wanted to fence off boundaries, interrupting trail access on the path's south side. A compromise was achieved, and the fence ended up being just below the trail area. A year later, the nonprofit Bonneville Shoreline Trail Committee was formed. Soon, legitimate access for the trail began to be approved in various other places too. By 1992, the University of Utah had agreed to allow an official corridor for the trail. Many legal access issues remain unresolved for stretches of the Bonneville Shoreline Trail, such as gaps in the path and a lack of safe access over busy roads, though bridges and tunnels have been added in places. The trail continues to mature, section by section.

This walk, above This Is the Place Heritage Park and the University of Utah's Research Park, may be the most difficult single path outlined in this book. However, the trek spans the key portion of the Bonneville Shoreline Trail that sparked the longer route's overall concept. At approximately 1,000 feet above the valley floor, the Shoreline Trail presents commanding views of the city and its valley, and it is quite accessible. Walkers, hikers, joggers, and bikers are allowed; technically, horses and dogs are not, on this segment, though you may well see some of the latter. Note that portions of the trail can be muddy after wet weather, and snowfall can make walking it inadvisable. Generally speaking, the trail's season of use is from late March to early November.

When you're through, if you have time, access to the towering, sculpture-festooned This Is the Place Monument nearby is free, as is This Is the Place Heritage Park's visitor center. The park's adjacent pioneer village requires a modest fee, and small passenger trains navigate its roadways, for those tired of walking. In addition, Hogle Zoo is right across the street.

● **Begin this walk at a signed trailhead, opposite and to the north of Hogle Zoo's parking lot, at approximately 2600 E. Sunnyside Ave. The small lot can accommodate perhaps a half dozen vehicles. Additional vehicles can park along Sunnyside to the west. Be sure to carry water. Note that the Shoreline Trail—especially in this area— involves a maze of spur trails that divide along the foothills, some diverting into adjacent canyons and clefts. However, other than delving west onto private property or actually walking up a side canyon to the east, there's little chance of getting lost. Walk through the gate and take one of two paths heading up the hill. Both paths subsequently merge. Be forewarned as well that this is a steep dirt trail at the beginning. Also, mountain bikers use the trail: Be vigilant, as bicyclists rarely stop for walkers.**

● **Passing a gully and old picnic tables and woodpiles, the trail temporarily levels out. Then it gets steep again, but you soon will be rewarded with sweeping views of the Salt Lake Valley, only oak brush and small trees popping up occasionally to block the perspective. The trail climbs about 340 vertical feet from the trailhead. Head north** along the mountainside. To make a loop walk possible, keep mostly to the winding trails on the right (east), hugging the hillside.

● Continue north, as the trail moderates. At the 0.5-mile mark, you will cross beneath power lines. The historic buildings of This Is the Place Heritage Park pose picturesquely below. Many are actual pioneer homes and structures relocated to this site, near where the first Mormon pioneers entered the Salt Lake Valley in 1847 via Emigration Canyon; others are replicas. At 0.8 mile, it may seem odd to see the miniature ship sitting on dry ground below. It represents pioneers who, instead of crossing the Great Plains, sailed around Cape Horn to the San Francisco area before coming to what was to become Utah. As signs note, the Shoreline Trail is following an easement above the park. Access is not permitted into the village from here, and cycling or jogging through Old Deseret Village is prohibited.

● To traverse a deep ravine, descend the trail, and then climb back out. At the 1-mile mark are portions of an old rail fence. In another 0.1 mile a gate marks the end of the Shoreline Trail's This Is the Place Heritage Park easement and the start of the University of Utah's Bonneville Trail segment. In spring, wildflowers dot the hillside. In high summer, despite drying grasses, butterflies and bees inspect remaining blossoms, and dragonflies—often called "darning needles"—miraculously float and dart through the air. Signs indicate the route of a buried natural gas pipeline (and, in fact, many call this the Pipeline Trail). At times, you will notice other parallel trails or even a dirt road below. Those will comprise part of your return route, creating a loop for this walk.

Along the Bonneville Shoreline Trail

- At almost 1.5 miles, the eastern path is significantly higher than its western tracks. The trail also returns to sections of oak brush, and at one point you will encounter a small section of rock steps. The University of Utah campus, Fort Douglas, and the University Medical Center campus come into clear view to the west and northwest. At 1.7 miles, the trail is directly above the Natural History Museum of Utah, the new Rio Tinto Center, distinguished by its copper paneling. That large open-pit operation visible to the southwest, in the Oquirrh Mountains? Rio Tinto's Bingham Canyon Mine.

- At the 1.85-mile mark, Red Butte Garden comes into view below, just north of the Rio Tinto Center. The hillside conservation garden and arboretum is a popular walking, touring, picnicking, and concert site. There is an entry fee. This is also the shoreline walk's turnaround point, when you encounter a faded trail-map sign. Now you can either take the trail that goes left and heads southwest down the hill, eventually reaching the lower-elevation trail segment, or you can backtrack for a half mile until you can more clearly spot a shorter connecting route to the lower paths.

- As you walk the lower path, it is often more like a wide dirt road. Both the trail-hugging eastern route and this path eventually funnel through the gate heralding reentry into This Is the Place Heritage Park territory. The lower trail offers closer views of the historic park's old pioneer buildings. The low path is generally more level and less serpentine than the upper trail, as well.

- Soon you will again see Sunnyside Ave. and Hogle Zoo. As you approach the parking area, choose which fork you want to take down the final steep portion to the roadside lot. This is a popular trail, and you will likely be able to ask other walkers and hikers for additional directions, if needed.

POINTS OF INTEREST (start to finish)

Hogle Zoo hoglezoo.org, 2600 E. Sunnyside Ave., 801-582-1631

Natural History Museum of Utah/Rio Tinto Center nhmu.utah.edu, University of Utah Research Park, 801-581-4303

Red Butte Garden redbuttegarden.org, 300 Wakara Way, University of Utah Research Park, 801-585-0556

This Is the Place Heritage Park thisistheplace.org, 2601 E. Sunnyside Ave., 801-582-1847

route summary

1. Begin this walk at a signed trailhead, opposite and to the north of Hogle Zoo's parking lot, at approximately 2600 E. Sunnyside Ave., on the north side of the street.

2. Walk through the gate and take one of two paths heading up the hill.

3. A maze of paths crisscross the area. Walk north, keeping to the east, hugging the hillside, and avoid diversions into side canyons.

4. Continue north as the trail moderates. At the 0.5-mile mark, the path goes under power lines. Avoid going too far west; fences mark the boundaries of This Is the Place Heritage Park, a fee area.

5. At 1.1 miles, you will reach a gate. This marks the end of This Is the Place's easement and the start of the University of Utah's Bonneville Trail segment.

6. At the 1.85-mile mark the Natural History Museum of Utah and Red Butte Garden are below. Red Butte is a fee area. This is this route's turnaround point, when you encounter a faded trail-map sign.

7. Now, you can either take a trail that goes left and heads southwest down the hill, eventually reaching the lower-elevation trail segment, or you can backtrack for a half mile until you can more clearly spot a shorter connecting route to the lower path.

8. Both trails will reconnect and funnel through the gate marking a return to This Is the Place Heritage Park territory.

9. Sunnyside Ave. and Hogle Zoo appear to the south. Choose which fork you want to take down the trail's final steep portion to the parking lot. Considering choosing the path you did not use to climb the hill from the lot.

10. Pass through the gate and return to the parking lot, where the Bonneville Shoreline Trail walk and hike began.

connecting the walks

Connect with Walk 20, This Is the Place, which begins a few hundred yards away, at This Is the Place Heritage Park.

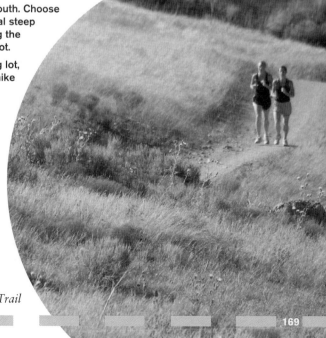

On the Bonneville Shoreline Trail

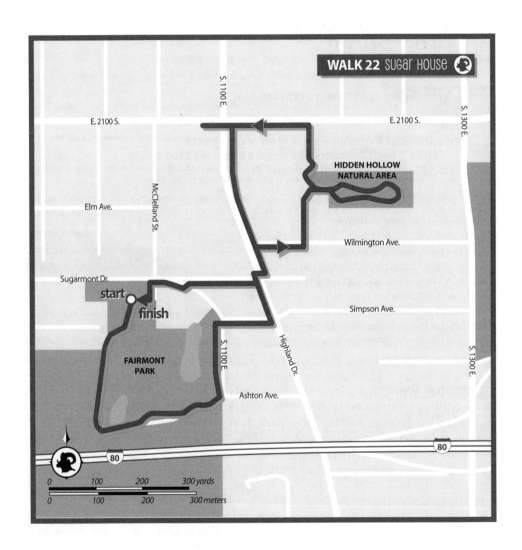

WALK 22 sugar house

E. 2100 S.

E. 2100 S.

S. 1100 E.

S. 1300 E.

HIDDEN HOLLOW
NATURAL AREA

Elm Ave.

McClelland St.

Wilmington Ave.

Sugarmont Dr.

start

finish

Simpson Ave.

S. 1100 E.

Highland Dr.

S. 1300 E.

FAIRMONT
PARK

Ashton Ave.

80

80

0   100   200   300 yards

0   100   200   300 meters

22 Sugar House: Sweet Dreams and Honored Beets

BOUNDARIES: 2100 South, 1300 East, I-215, 1000 East
DISTANCE: 2.3 miles
DIFFICULTY: Easy
PARKING: Free parking at Fairmont Park and on many streets
PUBLIC TRANSIT: Utah Transit Authority bus route #21 serves 2100 South; bus route #220 operates along Highland Dr.

Despite its pleasant name, nary a single cube of sugar was made in the residential and commercial neighborhood called Sugar House. This southeast section of Salt Lake City got its start in 1853, and an early dream was to indeed produce sugar here. Sugar was a rare commodity in pioneer times, and the settlers' answer was not sugarcane, but the sugar beet. A test factory was constructed and equipment shipped from Liverpool, England, but a sugar mill never materialized. Instead, the facility became a paper mill.

And talk about exchanging sweet for sour: Sugar House was, for many decades, home to the territorial and state prisons. A vibrant commercial district evolved, though, second only to the city's downtown. Furniture stores, for some reason, were a dominant enterprise. And the district became, and remains, a place of parks. Sprawling Sugar House Park, on land donated by the state in the early 1950s and occupying the former prison site, blankets hills and vales along Emigration Creek. But part of the community's original park, Hidden Hollow, fell into oblivion—until its resurrection in the 1990s. (Check out this chapter's Back Story.) Nearby Fairmont Park has roots in another older park, Forest Dale, "reclaimed and built" in 1935 by the Depression-era Works Progress Administration, bronze plaques note. The Forest Dale name remains attached to a city golf course to the south, separated from Fairmont by a freeway. The golf course, which opened in 1905, is Utah's oldest.

Sugar House possesses the distinct ambience of a busy crossroads community, a flavor that gives it an identity separate from its parent, Salt Lake City. A 55-foot-tall obelisk and attendant statuary, at 1100 E. 2100 South, celebrate pioneer history. Quaint Sprague Library seems the very epitome of a small-town haven for children and other book lovers. The business district has expanded, though empty historic lots seem to cry out for better times and a revival.

And then there are the beets. During a stroll through the heart of Sugar House you're bound to come across massive sugar beet sculptures scattered about several locations. Even legendary Jack, of giant beanstalk fame, might marvel at these bronze tributes to an underappreciated plant.

- Begin this walk in Salt Lake City's Fairmont Park, near the intersection of Sugarmont Dr. and McClelland St. (about 2245 South and 1045 East). The 30-acre park is open 5 a.m.–11 p.m. Take a stroll around the center of this L-shaped park by walking south on a path among its picnic areas. Soccer fields and a skateboard park occupy the southwest section. Veer left (east) and head for the center flagpole. A plaque on it, courtesy of the American Legion, quotes a 13th-century prayer of Saint Francis of Assisi, asking, "Lord, make me an instrument of your peace."

- Walk east toward the park's pond, where ducks, geese, and other aquatic birds mingle. The large, modern building at the pond's north end is Salt Lake County's Fairmont Aquatics Center, with a swimming pool, lap pool, and other amenities.

- Walk east to 1100 East, exiting on the park's east side. Turn left and walk north to Simpson Ave. (2222 South). Turn right and walk east though this area of small businesses to major Highland Dr. Proceed north on Highland Dr. to Sugarmont Dr. Turn right, cross Highland Dr. to the street's east side, and walk a few hundred feet north to Wilmington Ave.

- Turn right and walk east up Wilmington, a main artery of the Sugar House Commons retail area.

- After only a few hundred feet, turn left and walk northeast into the large retail parking lot. A discount movie theater is farther up Wilmington Ave. A Big 5 sports store and a Wendy's restaurant are nearby. Among the many stores is a Sundance Catalog Outlet, an upscale store one might expect to find nearer the resorts of Park City than in Sugar House. There is also a Whole Foods Market.

- Visually locate an arch near the Petco store in the northeast corner of the parking lot serving this retail cornucopia, for this is your next destination. Walk to and under the arch. A sky-blue city-parks sign bids you welcome to a near-secret park, Hidden Hollow Natural Area, also open 5 a.m.–11 p.m.

● Walk east along Parley's Creek, remaining on the stream's south side, the beginning of a Hidden Hollow loop. Nature and historical markers line the path. The Fredrick P. Sandberg Memorial Bridge crosses the creek. It is worth a pause here to gaze into and along the stream. As the natural area's signs note, Hidden Hollow boasts a half dozen different plant zones: a maple grove, a riparian forest, marsh wetland, an oak grove, foothill shrub and grass, and a pinyon-juniper grove. A loop through Hidden Hollow gives you a chance to stroll through all six, and signs decorated with children's drawings of creatures such as a meadow mouse, a robin, and a katydid, tell all about the water, trees, plants, and animals.

● Continue walking east through Hidden Hollow on either the concrete path on the south side of the stream or on a footpath a little farther south on the hillside. Both trails converge on the little park's east side, where you will spot a leafy example of Sugar House's (dare we say unique?) way-larger-than-life sugar beet sculptures. Artist Day Christensen's cast-bronze works pay affectionate tribute to the community's pioneer and farming roots. Stairs to the east lead to office buildings and 1300 East, which are not our goal.

● You've crossed Parley's Creek, so turn left, walking briefly north, and continue as the path turns to dirt and curves west, on a hillside above the stream's north side. The path may be muddy at times here. If so, reverse course and walk back to the west end of Hidden Hollow via the paved paths. Otherwise, continue west on the dirt trail. A Homestead

Sprague Library

173

Back Story

What can schoolchildren accomplish in their community? A great deal, if you look back at the rebirth and success of Sugar House's Hidden Hollow Natural Area.

Hidden Hollow, once part of the original Sugar House Park in the early 20th century, might not exist today were it not for the initiative and dreams of a group of Hawthorne Elementary School students in 1990. They rediscovered a forlorn three-acre spot along Parley's Creek engulfed by retail and commercial enterprises and buildings. As KOPE—Kids Organized to Protect Our Environment—they lobbied local government and businesses to save it. The students, joined by children from other schools, also helped clean up decades' worth of accumulated garbage and construction debris so that more people might share their vision of what the urban hollow could become.

As early as 1991, the KOPE kids were honored by President George H. W. Bush with the President's Environmental Youth Award. By 2000—with a master plan emphasizing nature; a conservation easement; new bridges; pathways; and nine years of hard work—the once-forgotten minipark had become a pleasant and popular destination once again. Today Hidden Hollow is a natural classroom, drawing scores of people out for a daily walk or jog and hosting a concert series each summer. Proposals for the future include a tunnel pathway to connect it with Sugar House Park and the Parley's trail system to the east, currently blocked by traffic-laden 1300 East.

"The natural area has been restored as a community treasure and serves as an example of what can happen when we work together to solve problems," notes a placard that tells the story of the dream that energized Sugar House schoolchildren: Hidden Hollow.

Studio Suites hotel is just north of the trail. A marker points out the site's railroad past, for on this grade the Utah Central Railway once ferried passengers and goods up Parley's Canyon to Park City. A health note: Other signs warn of poison ivy.

● When you reach the side of a sushi restaurant, you are exiting Hidden Hollow on its west side. Look around, a little to the south, and note that there are two additional sugar beet sculptures nearby. You could easily reenter Hidden Hollow and do a slightly different walk, as it is only about a quarter mile around the paved trails and back. Upon exiting, walk north through the retail area and connect with 2100 South. The area includes various businesses, including clothing stores, restaurants, and a bookseller. Across 2100 South, and slightly to the northeast, is the old Irving School House, now an apartment complex that retains the stone-and-brick look of the 1926 junior high.

- Turn left and walk west down the hill along the south side of 2100 South. Some of Sugar House's more eclectic businesses are across the street, including coin, music, and sports consignment stores—and a surf shop.

- Continuing west, cross Highland Dr. to an intersection island with a bus stop, a sign featuring a large map of the Sugar House area, and Sugar House's signature obelisk. The towering monument, erected in 1930 and dedicated in 1934—at the height of the Great Depression—is graced by sculptural works by Millard Fillmore Malin. The stone-work is topped by two eight-foot-tall Indians, representing the area's Native American legacy. A sculpture of a striking young woman on the east pediment symbolizes the Salt Lake Valley's fruitfulness, while a muscular fellow on the west, a mill builder, represents industry. One placard details the importance of the original sugar beet fac-tory as a symbol of pioneer enterprise. Southwest of the island are more interesting business nooks—a characteristic of the district—including Rockwood Art Studios and Cobwebs Antiques and Collectibles.

- Return east to Highland Dr., crossing to the east side. Turn right and walk south down Highland Dr. In a few hundred yards is Sprague Library, with a history dating back to 1914. During library hours, take a quick peek inside the building, where the computer age and shelves of books comingle. Next door to the south is a white-linen banquet hall inhabiting the former Sugar House Post Office.

- Continue walking south on Highland Dr. to Sugarmont St. Turn right at this intersec-tion, cross Highland Dr., immediately cross Sugarmont to the other side, and head west down Sugarmont on its only sidewalk, on the street's south side. In about a half block you have returned to this route's starting point, Fairmont Park.

POINTS OF INTEREST (START TO FINISH)

Fairmont Park slcclassic.com/publicservices/parks/parkspages/Fairmont.htm,
  1040 E. Sugarmont Dr., 801-972-7800

Fairmont Aquatic Center recreation.slco.org/fairmont, 1044 East Sugarmont Dr.,
  801-486-5867

Sundance Catalog Outlet sundancecatalog.com, 2201 S. Highland Dr., 801-487-3400

Hidden Hollow Natural Area slcclassic.com/slcgreen/openspace/Hidden_Hollow.htm,
  1255 E. 2160 South, 801-972-7800

Rockwood Art Studios rockwoodartstudios.com, 1062 & 1064 E. 2100 South

Cobwebs Antiques and Collections 1054 E. 2100 South, 801-485-9295

Sprague Public Library slcpl.lib.ut.us, 2131 S. 1100 East, 801-594-8640

Forest Dale Golf Course slcclassic.com/publicservices/golf/ForestDale.html,
  2375 S. 900 East, 801-483-5420

ROUTE SUMMARY

1. Begin this walk in Fairmont Park, near the intersection of Sugarmont Dr. and McClelland St. Walk west through the center of this L-shaped park, then curve south.

2. Turn left (east) to the center flagpole. Continue east to the park's pond and beyond, to 1100 East, on the park's east side.

3. Turn left and walk north to Simpson Ave.

4. Turn right and walk east to Highland Dr.

5. Continue north on Highland Dr. to the Sugarmont Dr. intersection and turn right to cross to Highland Dr.'s east side.

6. Turn right and walk east up Wilmington. After a few hundred feet, turn left and walk northeast into the large retail parking lot, moving toward its northeast corner.

7. Walk under the arch in the lot's northeast corner and enter Hidden Hollow Natural Area.

8. Stroll south along Parley's Creek, eventually looping back to the west on either the dirt trail on the stream's north side or the paved trail.

9. Exit Hidden Hollow on its west side, turn right, and walk north through a retail area to connect with 2100 South.

10. Turn left and walk west down the hill along the south side of 2100 South.

11. Cross Highland Dr. to a large traffic island featuring the Sugar House obelisk.

12.   Return east to Highland Dr., crossing to the east side of the street.

13.   Turn right and walk south along Highland Dr. to Sugarmont Dr.

14.   Turn right, crossing Highland Dr., then turn left to cross Sugarmont Dr., and then right to proceed west along Sugarmont's south side, the only side with a sidewalk.

15.   In about a half block you have returned to the walk's starting point, Fairmont Park.

CONNECTING THE WALKS

Connect with Walk 23, Sugar House Park, directly to the east across 1300 East, with motor vehicle access off 2100 South.

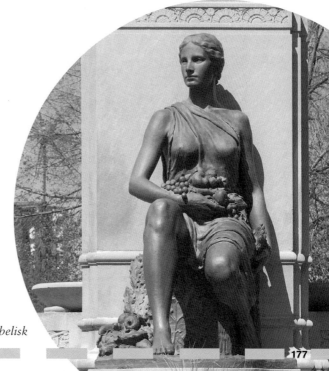

A sculpture on the Sugar House obelisk

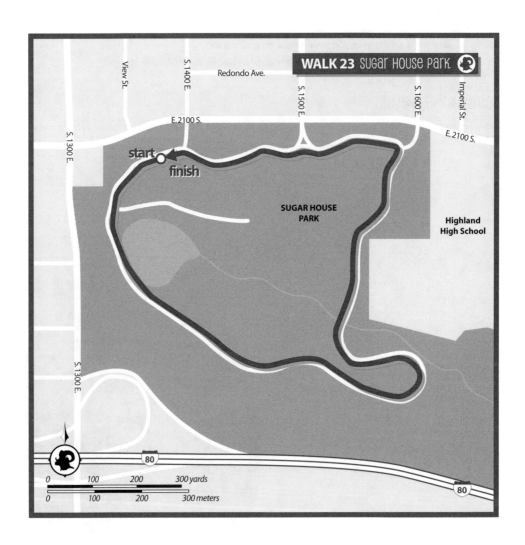

View St.

S. 1400 E.

Redondo Ave.

S. 1500 E.

S. 1600 E.

Imperial St.

E. 2100 S.

E. 2100 S.

S. 1300 E.

start

finish

SUGAR HOUSE PARK

Highland High School

S. 1300 E.

80

80

0   100   200   300 yards

0   100   200   300 meters

23 Sugar House Park: The City's Emerald Jewel

BOUNDARIES: 1300 East, 2100 South, Ram Blvd./1700 East, and I-215
DISTANCE: 1.4–2 miles
DIFFICULTY: Moderate
PARKING: Free in park
PUBLIC TRANSIT: Utah Transit Authority bus routes #21, 220, and 223 serve the area.

Occupying 110 acres of rolling creekside hill and valley, Sugar House Park is an emerald gem on Salt Lake City's southeast side, a welcome respite for many from the urban hustle and bustle right on its busy bordering streets. A 1.4-mile-loop road slinks through the park in a counterclockwise fashion, offering plenty of room for motorists, walkers, joggers, strollers, cyclists, and skateboarders. It is a huge space, where the only time you may ever feel crowded is on the sunniest of sunny weekend days or on a major summer holiday.

The park is named, of course, for the surrounding neighborhood, where Mormon pioneers first began their efforts to manufacture sugar from sugar beets. The park dates to the early 1950s, though it has been a historic location for a century and a half. You'd never know by looking at it now, but from 1854 to 1951 this pleasant, open place with few fences and walls, 6 miles from Salt Lake City's center, was Utah's territorial prison, operated by the federal government and, after statehood in 1896, the Utah State Prison.

Today it is one of the city's most popular pleasure grounds and offers great vistas of the nearby mountains. Sugar House Park encompasses two playgrounds, 10 pavilions, athletic fields, a garden center with a fine collection of rosebushes, and a four-acre pond, with Parley's Creek flowing through its center. Families picnic, hold reunions, fly kites, or simply stop to feed the birds by the pond. On the loop road, vehicular traffic must flow one way only, with a maximum speed of 20 mph. A yellow line on the loop's left side reserves a lane for nonmotorized travel, making it a popular exercise route. Others walk on the park's fringe sidewalk, for a route that is closer to 1.8 miles. Highland High School and its sports fields are on the park's eastern boundary.

Because it is so open, the park remains popular in winter, when joggers and walkers are joined by others using it as a miniature cross-country skiing course or screaming on sleds and tubes flying down a steep little hill in the park's southwest corner. Sugar House Park is open daily, 7 a.m.–10 p.m. in summer and 7 a.m.–9 p.m. in winter. Dogs are allowed in the park but must be leashed. No alcohol or smoking is allowed inside park boundaries.

- Enter Sugar House Park by heading east on 2100 South and turning right into the first entrance at 1400 East. If driving, turn right again on the loop road and park along the right side of the road. Begin your walk here. Walk counterclockwise on the left side of the road, inside the yellow line. You'll stroll downhill first, before looping south around the park's pond. Soon on your left will be a side road into the Big Field Pavilion and pond area.

- At the far south side of the pond, you can take this optional side route for another two or three tenths of a mile. If you opt to do this, turn left off the road and into the first picnic area, the Fabian Lakeside Pavilion. Enjoy the pond from a higher vantage, where many park-goers feed ducks, geese, and other birds. Seasonally, there are restrooms and drinking fountains available. Walk farther north to inspect Parley's Creek as it rushes (in spring) or meanders through the park's center. A small foot-bridge to the east safely traverses the stream in any season.

- Either return to the main loop road or continue along it, if you didn't take the side stroll. You will now be walking uphill and eastward and will pass by the park office, Sego Lilly Pavilion, and then Mount Olympus Pavilion, all on your right side. Then you will walk downhill and loop briefly westward before the serpentine road straightens and continues northward. Here is where you will also pass, on the right, the entrance to Hidden Grove Pavilion, the largest picnic area in the park. After the road straightens, you will also be along the western edge of Highland High School and will walk by the entrance to the Parley's Creek Pavilion, on your left.

- Now you will climb another hill on the loop road, heading northeast slightly before passing the Sugar House Garden Center, on the right. Here the looping road turns west for the final leg of this walk in the park. You will intersect the 1500 East exit from the park, where all vehicles must leave the park. Walkers can continue west to the 1400 East entrance.

- Want more exercise? Consider making a second loop, or wander and explore the park's wide-open grassy areas and hillocks.

POINTS OF INTEREST (START TO FINISH)

Sugar House Park Authority sugarhousepark.org, 801-467-1721

Highland High School highland.slcschools.org, 2166 S. 1700 East, 801-484-4343

Sugar House Garden Center 1610 E. 2100 South, 801-467-1721

ROUTE SUMMARY

1. Enter Sugar House Park via 2100 South, turning into the entrance at 1400 East and finding a place to park.

2. Walk counterclockwise on the left side of the road, inside the yellow line. You'll stroll downhill first, before swinging south around the park's pond.

3. At the far south side of the pond area, you can take an optional excursion toward the park's center for another two or three tenths of a mile. To do this, turn left off the road and into the first picnic area, and wander as you desire.

4. Either return to the loop road or continue along it, if you didn't take the side stroll. You will now be walking uphill and generally eastward.

5. Walk downhill and loop back westward, as the road straightens and continues northward.

6. As the winding paved road curves, climb another hill, heading slightly northeast.

7. Still on the road, loop west to begin the walk's final leg. You will intersect the 1500 East motor-vehicle exit from the park; continue walking west.

8. Pass the 1400 East park entrance, continuing to where your walk began.

9. If you wish, consider a second loop or a more leisurely exploration of the park.

CONNECTING THE WALKS

Connect with Walk 22, Sugar House, west of 1300 East on 2100 South.

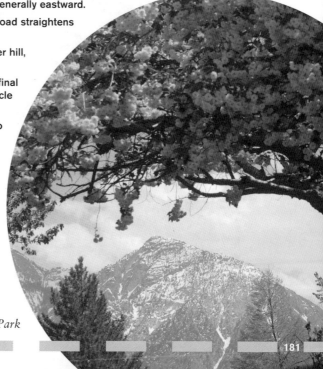

Mt. Olympus from Sugar House Park

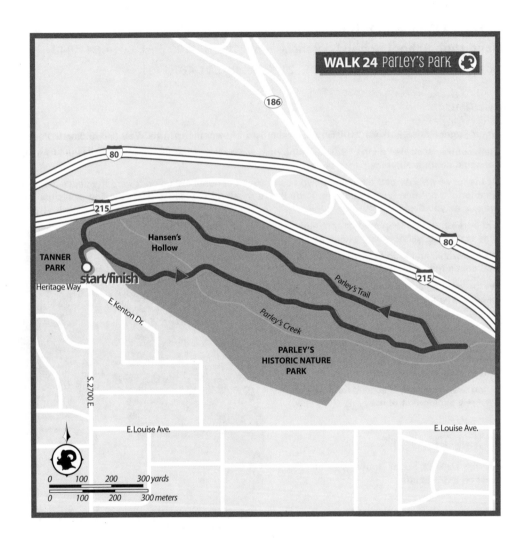

186

80

215

80

215

Hansen's
Hollow

Parley's Trail

Parley's Creek

**TANNER
PARK**

start/finish

Heritage Way

E. Kenton Dr.

S. 2700 E.

**PARLEY'S
HISTORIC NATURE
PARK**

E. Louise Ave.

E. Louise Ave.

0   100   200   300 yards

0   100   200   300 meters

24 Parley's Park: Nature and History in the Hollow

BOUNDARIES: I-80, I-215, 2300 East, and 2960 South
DISTANCE: 2 miles
DIFFICULTY: Moderate
PARKING: Free in Tanner Park, the trailhead, 2700 East and Heritage Way (2760 South)
PUBLIC TRANSIT: Utah Transit Authority bus route #223 serves 2300 South and 2700 East, several blocks from the trailhead.

Long ago, Hansen Hollow's depths bustled, in a fashion, with traffic. People on foot, on horseback, in wagons, in stagecoaches, and later on railroad trains moved through this crossroads at the mouth of Parley's Canyon. An inn, a brewery and saloon, farmsteads, a gravel pit, mills, and early rails all shared the hollow, one of the primary routes into and out of the Salt Lake Valley in the 19th century.

The low corridor has been superseded by superhighways. High above, the modern I-80 and I-215 freeways—titanic works of engineering, humming with heavy traffic—hem in the gulch. Who would expect that below foothill suburbs and these sculpted highways, a rough version of the valley's past can still be found in Parley's Historic Nature Park? To say the park is nature at its most pristine would be a stretch. Man's presence remains evident in the hollow—as does that of canines. Much of the park is an off-leash area for excited dogs and dog lovers, though great effort is expended to minimize what they might, um, leave behind. In addition, Rocky Mountain Power has an electrical substation at the western end, a few old car bodies litter the interior, BMX bike riders carved a challenging course in one section, and old byways and structures haunt the area.

Today, 88-acre Tanner Park covers a good portion of the hollow's south rim. It includes restrooms, as well as a playground, picnic areas, tennis courts, and a baseball field. Also nearby is the Jewish community's Congregation Kol Ami, west of Tanner Park. Prominently on the rim to the east is the headquarters building for the Sons of Utah Pioneers.

Harvey D. Hansen donated the original five acres needed to spark the beginnings of Parley's Historic Nature Park in 1979. Salt Lake City purchased another five acres from Hansen, and more land acquisition followed. The park was open, complete with trailside historic signs, by 1996. Parley's Nature Park trails are envisioned as part of a complex of valley-spanning pedestrian and bicycle routes. A northern path links to the paved Parley's Trail above. A mile to the southeast is the Parley's Crossing Trailhead at 3300 S. Wasatch Blvd., including two freeway-spanning bridges. The trail also connects to the Bonneville Shoreline Trail.

The noise of traffic overhead declines significantly upon walking down into Hansen Hollow from the parking area and trailhead in Tanner Park. Robins, bluejays, and smaller birds flock and chirp, taking splashy baths in available puddles, and the rippling waters of Parley's Creek calm the soul. You might just forget you are on the east side of the most populated valley in the Beehive State.

- Begin this counterclockwise loop through Parley's Historic Nature Park at the east edge of rim-top Tanner Park, at the junction of 2700 East and Heritage Way (2760 South). The best starting point is to walk to Heritage Way and 2700 East, though there is a short unmarked and unpaved trail on the parking lot's northeast corner. Signs note that dogs must be leashed in Tanner Park and its parking lot.

- Turn left to a gate, walking an initially paved path to enter Parley's Historic Nature Park. Asphalt wanes. Follow the trail's curving right fork downhill. Signs advise visitors to follow leash laws and to clean up after their canine companions. Plastic bags and "poop pipes" are provided for storage. Surprisingly, freeway noise diminishes rapidly as you descend into the hollow. Birds abound, and box elder, scrub oak, and cottonwood trees begin to dominate.

- Walk east on the widest path. In Hansen Hollow's bottomland, 0.5 mile out, cross a bridge over Parley's Creek. Exercise caution around this water, especially during spring runoff season. The path soon opens even wider, with only the occasional glimpse of a home or building sitting on the rim above, or the faint whoosh of I-80 and I-215 to remind you of nearby civilization.

- At 0.7 mile from Tanner Park, you will reach your first sitting bench. Fork right here, as the left fork leads to the paved Parley's Trail higher up the hill. Another hundred feet farther along is a plaque on a boulder honoring Harvey D. Hansen, who donated land for the park. In a few hundred more feet is another boulder plaque, honoring John J. "Jack" Nielsen, a key volunteer in developing the nature park.

- Parley's Creek soon courses along the right side of the path. You may also notice a small footbridge on the right, which leads uphill to the neighborhood on the south rim. Parley's Creek was originally called Big Kanyon Creek. Its name was changed after enterprising pioneer Parley P. Pratt surveyed the canyon for a toll road (also nicknamed "The Golden Pass Road"). Pratt's toll road opened on July 4, 1850, only three years after settlers entered the Salt Lake Valley, and meant future immigrants and travelers could avoid the grueling Big and Little Mountain climbs in Emigration Canyon. The original toll for the road was 75 cents for a two-horse outfit and 10 cents for each additional pack or saddle animal; sheep were a penny per head. Today, I-80 barrels through Parley's Canyon.

- Continue southeast as the hollow narrows. Parts of the dirt road you have followed roughly correspond to the original pioneer approach road to Parley's Canyon. Do not cross a second footbridge. At 1 mile out, you will be able to see cars to the east traveling I-215. Remain to the left, by the fence line.

- After another several hundred feet, you will see another commemorative sign on a rock, to "The Railroad," which steamed through the area in pioneer mining days. By the late 1870s, a railroad connected Salt Lake City to Coalville, to the east, through Parley's Canyon. Soon after, a spur was added to Park City, best known for its rich silver mines. The last train chugged through the hollow on January 5, 1956. You will soon see the end of the hollow, where a bench overlooks where Parley's Creek is funneled here through a conduit under the freeway.

- Turn around and retrace your path a few hundred feet, looking for a path that goes right and uphill to the northeast toward the paved Parley's Trail. Walk this route as it follows a wood fence. Turn left and walk northwest on the paved trail. This asphalt path has two lanes. Remain on the right side and be vigilant for fast-moving bicycles, although their posted speed limit is 20 mph. You are headed west.

- At 1.25 miles out is a historic marker for the Golden Pass Road and Toll House. Soon after, the trail temporarily becomes cement. Look for a plaque identifying Dudler's

Wine Cellar. The sign will be on the right, about 200 feet off the trail. A hotel was operated in the area from 1864 to 1897, serving travelers going up and down Parley's Canyon. Yes, homemade liquor was served here to travelers—despite the area's strong Mormon influence—at what was known as Dudler's Tavern. It was owned by the Shear (Schaer) family. Vandals burned what was left of the inn in 1952. To the right (north) here, you will see a gated cave. This is the old wine cellar. Unfortunately, graffiti is everywhere.

● Return to the paved path and continue west. In another quarter mile you will see a sandstone arch to the right (north). The graffiti-marked stonework is what remains of a pioneer aqueduct. Native Americans, plaques note, called Parley's Creek "Obit-ko-ke-che."

● Walk another quarter mile along Parley's Trail and you will reach an area of newly planted trees on the right and will spot an old truck bed on the left. The final 440 yards of the trail will include some short 9% grades up and down. Also nearby is an electrical substation, on the left side below. Along the last 200 yards, the trail parallels the noisy freeway and is on the same level as the road as it climbs back to Tanner Park, the walk's starting point.

POINTS OF INTEREST (start to finish)

Parley's Historic Nature Park/Tanner Park Trailhead slcclassic.com/publicservices/parks/Parleys/parleysnaturepark.htm, 2700 East and Heritage Way

Congregation Kol Ami conkolami.org, 2425 Heritage Way, 801-484-1501

Sons of Utah Pioneers Building sonsofutahpioneers.org, 3301 E. 2920 South (on the rim at the southeast side of Parley's Hollow), 866-724-1847

route summary

1. Begin this counterclockwise loop at the east edge of Tanner Park, 2700 East and Heritage Way (2760 South).

2. Turn left and walk a few hundred feet to a gate at the end of 2700 East, and enter Parley's Historic Nature Park.

3. Walk southeast and downhill, choosing the dirt path on the right and not the paved trail to the north.

4. Keep walking southeast and cross a bridge 0.5 mile from the start.

5. Turn right at 0.7 mile, near a park bench.

6. Do not cross a second bridge here, but keep heading for the end of the hollow to the southeast.

7. At the end of the hollow is a bench overlooking a conduit where Parley's Creek enters Hansen's Hollow. Turn around and look for a trail to the northwest.

8. Take the side trail that leads to the paved Parley's Trail uphill. Turn left at the two-lane pedestrian and bicycle path and walk northwest.

9. Follow the path around Hansen Hollow's west side, turning south and up to Tanner Park, the walk's starting point.

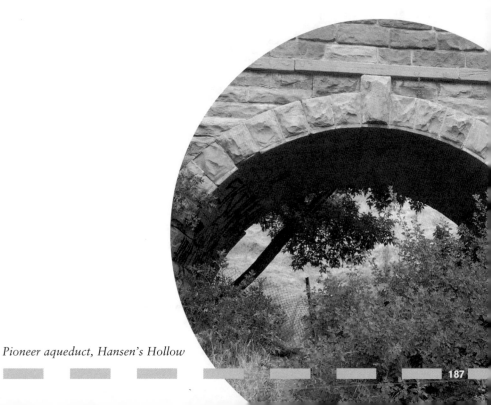

Pioneer aqueduct, Hansen's Hollow

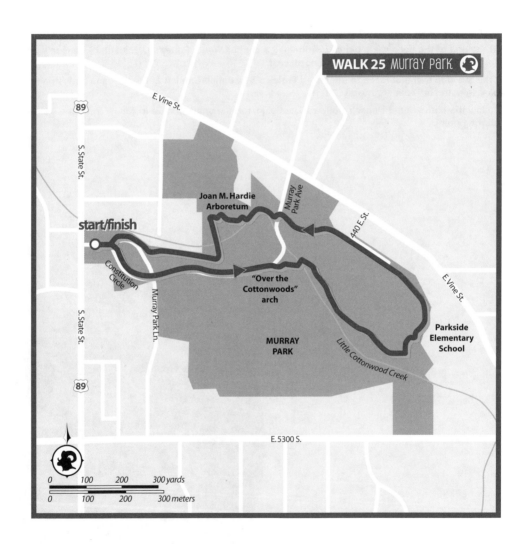

WALK 25 Murray Park

E. Vine St.

89

S. State St.

Joan M. Hardie Arboretum

Murray Park Ave

440 E. St.

start/finish

Constitution Circle

Murray Park Ln.

"Over the Cottonwoods" arch

E. Vine St.

MURRAY PARK

Little Cottonwood Creek

Parkside Elementary School

89

E. 5300 S.

0   100   200   300 yards
0   100   200   300 meters

Murray Park: Oasis in the Center of it All

BOUNDARIES: **State St., Vine St./4940 South, and 5300 South**
DISTANCE: **1.5 miles**
DIFFICULTY: **Easy**
PARKING: **Free parking inside the park**
PUBLIC TRANSIT: **Utah Transit Authority bus route #200 runs from 5300 South and State St. in Murray to downtown Salt Lake City; UTA's TRAX light-rail's Murray Central Station is west of the park, across State St. and behind the Intermountain Medical Center**

Murray City dubs itself "the hub" of the Salt Lake Valley, as it is in the valley's center. In turn, at the core of this hub is a pleasant urban refuge: Murray Park. This green space, which serves a community of almost 50,000 residents (and many others besides), is 6 miles south of downtown Salt Lake City proper. One of the metropolitan area's busiest arteries, State St., is the park's western entry and boundary. Across the way is the region's newest multi-disciplinary health-care flagship, Intermountain Medical Center. Murray Park's sometimes tree-canopied, occasionally rolling 36-plus acres parallel Little Cottonwood Creek. Founded, as one marker notes, in 1924, the walk-friendly park provides a stark contrast to the busy streets and the commercial and medical hubbub so close by. The park has picnic areas with grills, five pavilions, playgrounds, and athletic fields. Its pluses include an amphitheater, an outdoor aquatic center, a rose garden, an arboretum, and an indoor multipurpose gymnasium. Salt Lake County operates an ice rink, used as practice space during Salt Lake's 2002 Winter Olympic Games.

Murray has always had an identity separate from both the nearby metropolis of Salt Lake City and the quilt of other communities surrounding it. For instance, while the schools in other valley communities are part of large school districts, most of Murray is served by the city's own compact district, funneling students to Murray High School, a few blocks south of Murray Park. As the city grew in recent years, it added neighborhoods served by another district, and thus Cottonwood High School to the east is also now in Murray. Other services, such as police, fire, and even electric power, are managed by the small city. Farming settlements were founded in the area in the middle of the 19th century, and the first post office bore the name South Cottonwood. "Murray" gained traction in 1883, when the growing town was named in honor of Civil War General Eli Murray, who was Utah's 12th territorial governor. The Pony Express passed through the village, as did migrating pioneers and even an army. As the century progressed, mining began to flourish in the Oquirrh Mountains to the west and the Wasatch Mountains to the east. Murray's central location offered handy railroad access. An ore smelting, sampling, and refining boom followed, and Murray became a key producer of refined silver, lead, copper, gold, and zinc—muscular industries that have since faded away entirely.

Murray's old downtown lines State St. to the north, but over the years other mercantile trends pulled business south of the park. The city's centrality began to attract automobile dealerships, and Murray is also home to one of the valley's principal malls, Fashion Place, at 6400 S. State St. And finally, in 2000, towering but unused smelter smokestacks that had long stood as Murray's highly visible landmarks west of the park were imploded to make way for today's Intermountain Medical Center.

In the midst of all this, Murray Park remains an oasis. The park is open during daylight hours and until 11 p.m. Dogs must be on a leash. Maps on pedestals at key points scattered throughout the park help visitors know just where they are.

- Enter Murray Park via its west entrance, at 5130 S. State St. You are at the park's small Constitution Circle loop. If in a vehicle, park along the road's right side; if no space is available, drive farther east to one of several nearby parking lots. Begin the walk near the park's west entrance. Note the huge tree-trunk carving of Chief Wasatch facing State St. A rose garden surrounding a colonaded pergola and plaza is to the right, on the entryway's south side. This part of the park was designated in 1950 as a war memorial and Garden of Freedom. In the small loop's center are two old military gun mounts, a flagpole, and a Vietnam War memorial.

- Walk east along Constitution Circle to connect with the park's sidewalk, running to the right side of some restrooms. When you reach a stop sign, carefully cross north-south Murray Park Lane, and continue walking east on east-west Murray Park Ave. A gazebo is on your left, and The Park Center indoor multipurpose facility and its parking lot are on your right. Next on the right come a seasonal concession stand and the park offices.

- Continue east to the clever, ornamented *Over the Cottonwoods* arch, hovering above the park's interior avenue. The artwork arch, by William Littig and Paul Heath, is adorned with metallic icons representing Murray's historic landmarks—from buildings to towers and smokestacks—and commemorates Utah's 1996 statehood centennial. Turn right here, off the sidewalk, toward a footbridge across Little Cottonwood Creek, beyond the park's Pavilion #5 and a playground.

- Cross the bridge and turn right to walk southeast along the stream. Almost a half-mile from the walk's start, this is a particularly scenic area of the park. Covered with lawn, shaded by trees, and including a pond, the section seems like a golf course—without the golfers. The open area does attract rambunctious children, however—and a hillock offers a vantage to catch the wind for kite flying (though kites caught in nearby trees bear witness that some folks experience Charlie Brown–like mishaps). Another footbridge is off to the right, but do not cross it. The path dead-ends at the park amphitheater.

- Proceed to a parking lot, veering left to walk east between the lot and Pavilion #2 on the left. Parkside Elementary School and more playgrounds are due east. The park's southeastern entrance is nearby. On the sidewalk, loop to the northwest. Next up are sections of the park's Vita Course, a self-guided 10-station outdoor exercise area, with various stretching and muscle-strengthening segments. Farther along on the left are additional restrooms and Pavilion #4. You are now about one full mile out from the walk's start.

- After passing a parking lot on your right, carefully traverse a section of road (440 East), one of Murray Park's northern entrances, and proceed on the sidewalk between an outdoor swimming pool and Ken Price Baseball Field. With a parking lot on the left (south), cross another entry street, 330 East, and head toward the park's Joan M. Hardle Arboretum. A seasonal outdoor ice rink is also to the left. Stroll through the arboretum, with its maze of intertwining sidewalks. A nearby monument remembers the terrorist attacks of September 11, 2001. The Murray Boys and Girls Club is north-west of the arboretum.

- After enjoying the arboretum, exit left to walk south, meandering past a pine grove and heading toward a footbridge, and cross Little Cottonwood Creek. Intermountain Medical Center buildings again loom to the west. Before reaching the park's gazebo, turn right on a walkway that parallels the stream. Constitution Circle is just ahead, as is this walk's starting point.

Back Story

The craggy head of a symbolic American Indian, carved from a tree trunk, greets those accessing Murray Park via its main entrance at 5130 S. State St. The huge figure is one of a series of more than 70 such artworks, together called the "Trail of the Whispering Giants," by Peter "Wolf" Toth. Examples are found in all 50 states, parts of Canada, and in Toth's native Hungary. He completed the Murray carving in 1985, mainly using a chainsaw to create the figure from a dead cottonwood tree.

Murray's statue is called *Chief Wasatch*. It is 23 feet tall and weighs more than 17 tons. A plaque on its stone base notes, in part, that the work was created to "raise the nation's conscience to the plight of the first American(s) so they won't be forgotten,—but will remembered—in our minds and in our hearts. This statue is sculptured out of a giant cottonwood tree in honor of Utah Native Americans— Southern and Northern Ute, Southern Shoshone, Goshutes, Paiute, and Navajo."

Wasatch is a Ute Indian word meaning "mountain pass" or "low place in a high mountain," according to the Utah State Historical Society. It is the name of a prominent Utah mountain range, a dramatic portion of which forms the Salt Lake Valley's east side. There was a notable Shoshone Indian leader with a similar name: Chief Washakie. During the 19th century he interacted with people such as mountain man Jim Bridger and Mormon leader Brigham Young, was a friend to pioneers and settlers, and served as an Army scout. Chief Washakie lived a long life, from about 1806 to 1900, participated in many peace treaties, and is a key figure in both Utah and Wyoming history.

POINTS OF INTEREST (START TO FINISH)

Murray Park murray.utah.gov, 296 E. Murray Park Ave., 801-264-2614

The Park Center in Murray Park murray.utah.gov/index.aspx?nid=720, 202 E. Murray Park Ave., 801-284-4200

Salt Lake County Ice Center countyice.slco.org, 5201 S. Murray Park Lane, 801-270-7280

Murray Boys and Girls Club bgcsv.org, 244 Myrtle Ave., 801-284-4254

Intermountain Medical Center intermountainhealthcare.org/hospitals/imed,
5121 Cottonwood St., 801-507-7000

route summary

1. Begin at Murray Park's west entrance. Walk east along Constitution Cir. to connect with the main park sidewalk.

2. At a stop sign, carefully cross Murray Park Lane (160 East) and continue along Murray Park Ave. east into the park.

3. At the Over the Cottonwoods arch, which looms over the interior park road, veer right, off the sidewalk, toward a footbridge across Little Cottonwood Creek.

4. Cross the bridge and turn right to walk southeast along the stream.

5. Proceed between a parking lot, on the right, and Pavilion #2, on the left. Parkside Elementary School is due east.

6. Follow the sidewalk to loop northwest.

7. Cross 440 East, a northern park entry, and walk on the sidewalk between an outdoor swimming pool and a baseball field.

8. At 330 East, another north entrance, cross the road and continue toward the park's Joan M. Hardle Arboretum.

9. Exit the arboretum to the south, and cross a footbridge over Little Cottonwood Creek.

10. Before reaching the park's gazebo, turn right to follow the sidewalk along the stream, heading west.

11. Constitution Circle marks a return to the vicinity of this walk's starting point.

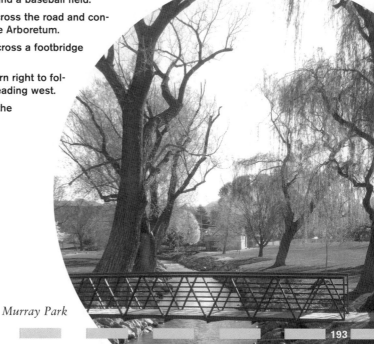

Murray Park

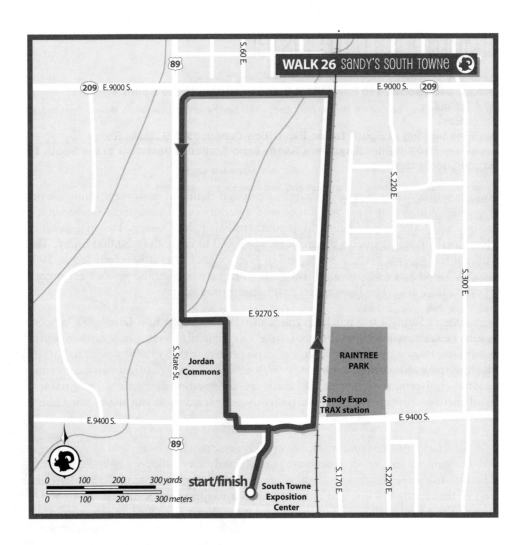

89
209 E. 9000 S.
S. 60 E.
E. 9000 S. 209

S. 220 E.

S. 300 E.

E. 9270 S.

RAINTREE
PARK

S. State St.

Jordan
Commons

Sandy Expo
TRAX station

E. 9400 S.

E. 9400 S.

S. 170 E.

S. 220 E.

89

0   100   200   300 yards
0   100   200   300 meters

start/finish

South Towne
Exposition
Center

26 SANDY'S SOUTH TOWNE: SALT LAKE'S AMBITIOUS LITTLE SISTER

BOUNDARIES: 9400 South, 150 East, TRAX light-rail line, and 9000 South
DISTANCE: 1.5 miles
DIFFICULTY: Easy
PARKING: Free parking at South Towne Exposition Center, 9575 S. State St.
PUBLIC TRANSIT: TRAX light-rail system's Sandy Expo Station is next door to the South Towne Exposition Center.

Through growth and development—hotels, a popular mall, entertainment venues, a professional soccer stadium (for Real Salt Lake), and a county exposition hall—Sandy City, Utah, has become Salt Lake City's little rival in southern Salt Lake County. The once-rural community blossomed from just over 6,000 residents in 1970 to more than 90,000 today. The proud nickname of the student body at local Jordan High School after it was founded in 1907? "The Beetdiggers." Students were released from school to help harvest the area's vital sugar beet crop. Today, they are "The Beetdiggers" still, and proud of it.

A cornerstone in Sandy's rise has been the South Towne Exposition Center, 9575 S. State St.—not to be confused with the South Towne Center mall, about a mile farther south. One of the busiest gathering places in Utah, the expo center, with 243,000 square feet of display and meeting space, hosts home, garden, gem, and auto shows; political party conventions; professional conferences; corporate and trade meetings; ethnic festivals . . . you name it— dozens of them each year. And it is conveniently connected to its big sister, Salt Lake City, 14 miles away via TRAX light-rail.

With almost four dozen restaurants, 1,200 hotel rooms, movie screens, and businesses galore in the vicinity, State St. and South Towne are part of Sandy City's modern hub. So, sometimes it might be nice to escape the crowds, right? One way to do that is to stroll the Sandy Rail Trail, just west of the nearby rail line and only 300 yards away from the South Towne Expo Center's front door. The paved path is part of the much longer Porter Rockwell Trail, named after a legendary gunslinger, a bodyguard to early Mormon leaders Joseph Smith Jr. and Brigham Young. The Sandy Rail Trail portion runs mostly parallel to the TRAX light-rail line. Promoted by the national Rails-to-Trails Conservancy, it is a straightforward, almost straight-line walk, with options to make a trek shorter or longer and to explore nearby Jordan Commons. (The full conservancy-promoted trail is 3 miles long, while the Porter Rockwell Trail continues to Draper to the south and stretches almost a dozen miles along an old railroad grade.)

Be aware that the first part of this route is along a sparsely shaded asphalt path. Most folks will want to avoid it during the heat of a summer's day. The trail is also popular with cyclists and in-line skaters.

- Head northeast from the South Towne Exposition Center to the Sandy Expo TRAX station at 150 E. 9400 South. Cross 9400 South at a pedestrian crossing directly west of the TRAX line. A path runs south and north, parallel to the TRAX line. It is a wide path, with a yellow line down its center; a fence on the east side separates it from the rail line.

- Walk north. The Jordan Commons entertainment and business district is on your left, notably represented by an office tower housing DeVry University and Oracle computer systems. A half mile out, the Sandy City Operations Center is on your left, followed soon by a corporate building and the Sandy City Fire Station.

- At 9000 South, turn left to walk west, as further northward progress is obstructed by the traffic pattern. There is no direct pedestrian crossing here to the Historic Sandy TRAX station across 9000 South. The only two pedestrian crossings are hundreds of yards away, to the west (State St.) or to the east (300 East). (If you do wish to continue north, see the options suggested below.)

- At State St., turn left to walk south on the east-side walkway, past automotive-related and other businesses. It is a slight uphill chug after a gradual descent along 9000 South. Across State St. to the west are the massive and distinctive white awnings of Rio Tinto Stadium, a 20,000-seat sports and entertainment venue that opened in 2008 as the home of Real Salt Lake. The professional Utah team won Major League Soccer's championship in 2009, and has had additional international success (by American standards) more recently.

- At 9270 South, cross to the street's south side and make a left turn to walk east. This is the north side of the Jordan Commons complex. The commercial center occupies the former site of Jordan High School and includes the Megaplex 17 movie theaters, restaurants, and office buildings.

- Jordan Commons' north-south traffic axis is at about 70 East. Turn right to walk south into the district's heart. Parking lots and terraces are on both sides of the street. The main entries to the theaters and the Commons' food court are on the right. At mid-block on the left is a cluster of popular sit-down restaurants to tempt your palate, including Ruby River Steakhouse, Joe's Crab Shack, and Last Samurai, a Japanese-themed grill and sushi bar.

- Continue south to 9400 South, where a pedestrian crosswalk and signal will return you to the South Towne Expo Center, where this walk began—though there are alternatives, if you want a longer walk or are interested in mixing in use of the handy TRAX line.

- One option would come at midtrek, at 9000 South, where you could walk east or west along this busy highway, crossing north at a signal. On the street's north side you could return to the Sandy Expo Station by riding TRAX or, a second possibility: The rail trail continues north once you've managed to ford the busy street. Older homes and Sandy's historic center and Main St. are in the neighborhood to the north.

- Yet another alternative, upon returning to 9400 South, is to walk along the south continuation of the Sandy Rail Trail, behind the Expo Center, to the Sandy Civic Center TRAX Station (10000 South), the end of the line. The modern Jordan High School campus, which looks more like a small college campus, lies west of this

Jordan Commons' restaurant and office areas

Back Story

As you stroll through Sandy, you will likely enjoy impressive views of the high, rugged Wasatch Mountains hulking to the east, especially when frosted in winter white. The range and its canyons are home to many of Utah's world-famous ski resorts (Alta, Snowbird, Brighton, Solitude, Sundance, Deer Valley, and The Canyons at Park City, among others) and are an outdoor recreation destination for local residents and visitors alike. Stretching from Soda Springs, Idaho, on the north, to Nephi, Utah, on the south, the Wasatch Front, the range's west flank, is home to most of Utah's almost three million residents.

In the Sandy area, the most prominent Wasatch summit is Lone Peak, so named for its westernmost prominence as viewed from the north, and the mountain's commanding presence over the southeastern Salt Lake Valley. Even though it juts a majestic 11,253 feet above sea level, Lone Peak is not the tallest in the Wasatch range. However, in Salt Lake County, only the American Fork Twin Peaks and Little Matterhorn Peak, behind Lone Peak, are taller.

Lone Peak is part of a wilderness area established in 1978. Hiking to its summit remains one of the area's top adventures, requiring a 14-mile round-trip hike that climbs some 6,000 vertical feet. Despite the distance and elevation gain, most trekkers do it in a single day. The topmost summit is exposed, as hikers are surrounded by cliffs and steep drop-offs. Lightning danger can be extreme, even deadly, during some summer days, when monsoonal clouds billow in the afternoons.

trail segment. This walk extension would add approximately 1.5 miles (for a walk total of 3 miles). An optional return, if you don't wish to retrace your steps, would be to ride TRAX back to 9400 South's Sandy Expo Station.

POINTS OF INTEREST (START TO FINISH)

South Towne Exposition Center southtowneexpo.com, 9575 S. State St., 801-565-4490

Utah Transit Authority's TRAX Sandy Expo Station rideuta.com, 150 E. 9400 South

Jordan Commons jordancommons.com, 9400 S. State St.

Utah Transit Authority's TRAX Historic Sandy Station rideuta.com, 165 E. 9000 South

Rio Tinto Stadium riotintostadium.com, 9256 S. State St., 801-727-2700

Megaplex 17 at Jordan Commons megaplextheatres.com, 9400 S. State St., 801-304-4577

Ruby River Steakhouse rubyriver.com, 85 E. 9400 South, 801-569-1885

Joe's Crab Shack joescrabshack.com, 65 E. 9400 South, 801-255-9571

Last Samurai lastsam.com, 95 E. 9400 South, 801-568-2888

Utah Transit Authority's TRAX Sandy Civic Center Station rideuta.com, 115 E. Sego Lily Dr. (10000 South)

South Towne Center southtownecenter.com, 10450 S. State St., 801-572-1516

route summary

1. Walk northeast from the South Towne Exposition Center toward the Sandy Expo TRAX station, 150 E. 9400 South. Cross 9400 South at a designated pedestrian crossing, directly west of the TRAX line.

2. Walk north on the asphalt trail that parallels the TRAX rail line to 9000 South.

3. At 9000 South, turn left to walk west to State St.

4. At State St., turn left to walk south to 9270 South, crossing to the south sidewalk.

5. On the corner, turn left and walk to about 70 East, the central north-south traffic corridor for Jordan Commons.

6. Turn right to walk south through the theater and commercial complex to 9400 South.

7. Cross 9400 South at a marked and signaled pedestrian walk.

8. You've returned to the South Towne Expo Center, where this walk began.

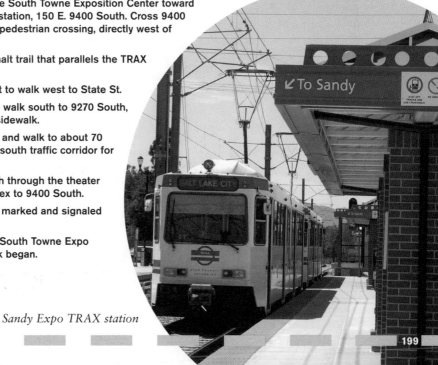

Sandy Expo TRAX station

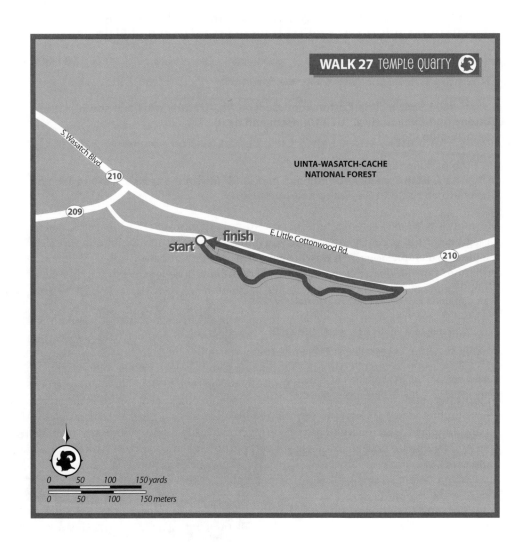

WALK 27 TEMPLE QUARRY

S. Wasatch Blvd.

UINTA-WASATCH-CACHE
NATIONAL FOREST

210

209

start

finish

E. Little Cottonwood Rd.

210

0   50   100   150 yards
0   50   100   150 meters

27 Temple Quarry: Taking the Mountains for Granite

BOUNDARIES: 9400 South/Little Cottonwood Canyon Rd. (UT 209; west and south), Little Cottonwood Canyon Hwy. (UT 210; north and east)
DISTANCE: 0.25-mile loop
DIFFICULTY: Easy
PARKING: Free parking lot
PUBLIC TRANSIT: A Utah Transit Authority bus park-and-ride lot is across UT 210 to the northwest. Buses are en route to Snowbird and Alta resorts.

The Mormons' Salt Lake Temple, built over a 40-year span, from 1853 to 1893, has to be considered one of the premier 19th-century manmade landmarks in the Intermountain West. The temple and Temple Square in downtown Salt Lake City are also Utah's number one tourist destination. But the question may arise: Where did all those massive granitelike blocks used to build the spired, and inspiring, edifice originate?

The answer: Temple Quarry, or nearby, at the mouth of Little Cottonwood Canyon, about 20 miles southeast of Salt Lake City. A visit to the quarry and boulder field, a history-nature trail created in 1993, gives almost everyone the opportunity for a short, refreshing walk away from the city, yet one that isn't a mountain hike or clamber. Interpretive signs outline the process of cutting and then hauling granite blocks to the temple site. There are restrooms and an amphitheater, and the trail itself is accessible to the handicapped, not to mention the little ones. Surrounding views are majestic, to say the least: sheer gray cliffs on either side of the canyon are popular rock-climbing destinations, yet are easily admired in safety from below. In spring and beyond, waterfalls cascade off certain notches and courses. At times, mountain goats and other wildlife pop into view. The Salt Lake Valley is framed to the west, and the view up-canyon emphasizes the power of Ice Age glaciers that carved its U shape.

Note that dogs are not allowed on Little Cottonwood Canyon trails, as this is a valley watershed. And consider the Temple Quarry Trail an introduction: The quarry trailhead is also the beginning of the longer Little Cottonwood Canyon Trail (about 3 miles one way), or a glance up Little Cottonwood Canyon may just lure you to drive farther east for more alpine scenery gawking and perhaps a visit to Snowbird or Alta ski and summer resorts.

● The trailhead is just south of the junction of UT 210 (Wasatch Blvd. to the northwest, which becomes the road up Little Cottonwood Canyon) and UT 209 (9400 South to the west, and Little Cottonwood Canyon Rd. here), near the canyon mouth. Watch for an open gate and a sign that pretty much says it all: "Temple Quarry Trailhead." Open daily, 7 a.m.–10 p.m., the trail is usually accessible from May to October each year, though snowshoers also use it in winter. After parking in the paved lot, walk east, where a loop path begins.

● Walk east, where a sign notes that the quarry began operation in 1861, in a debris field of huge boulders. "History has left its mark on Little Cottonwood Canyon," one historic marker notes. "In the late 1880s and early 1900s this was a busy place! Mining, lumbering and quarrying drew hundreds, even thousands, of people to towns that have since died. Graniteville, Wasatch, Hoggum, Tannersville, Central City . . ., and Emmaville are gone, but the stories and evidence of occupation remain." The first temple stones were laboriously moved using ox teams and wagons. After the railroad came to Utah in 1869, a route was brought to Sandy in the valley below, and then a line was extended to the quarry in 1873. That made hauling the rough-cut stones much simpler.

● As you continue east on the loop, be sure to look up at the quartz monzonite of the rugged canyon walls, the stuff from which the temple blocks were made. Quartz monzonite is a variety, or close relative, of granite. It is an intrusive igneous rock, which forms when magma is forced into areas underground and cools. This quarry's quartz monzonite is commonly known as temple granite, or white granite, a marker notes. It is familiar to Utahns from use in the temple and other structures, and because of its salt-and-pepper appearance and the sparkle of embedded mica. Redwood benches are available along the path for those who wish to pause, ponder, or rest.

● At just over 0.1 mile along the path, take a right turn to visit one of the massive boulders left behind by the temple builders. Many such rocks still bear chisel marks and cuts. At 0.16 mile is another mountain viewpoint and another redwood bench. Stands of oak brush provide shade as the trail curves and loops west.

● The loop returns to the parking lot, completing this short, exploratory mountain walk. An optional, much longer trail, which partially follows the old railroad bed, also begins at the eastern end of the parking lot. The rough and rocky Little Cottonwood Canyon Trail, popular with both hikers and mountain bikers, continues 3 miles up the canyon. The dirt path climbs 1,090 vertical feet and offers views of Lisa Falls.

POINTS OF INTEREST (START TO FINISH)

Alta Ski Resort alta.com, 801-359-1078

Snowbird Ski and Summer Resort snowbird.com, 800-232-9542

ROUTE SUMMARY

1. Start at the Temple Quarry Trailhead, at the junction of UT 209 and UT 210. The former is an extension of 9400 South; the latter is an extension of Wasatch Blvd., as it becomes the main canyon road.

2. Begin the loop trail at the west end of the parking lot, just past the restrooms.

3. Turn right on a side trail to a large boulder and viewpoint.

4. After just 0.25 mile, the trail loops west, returning to the parking lot, where this walk began.

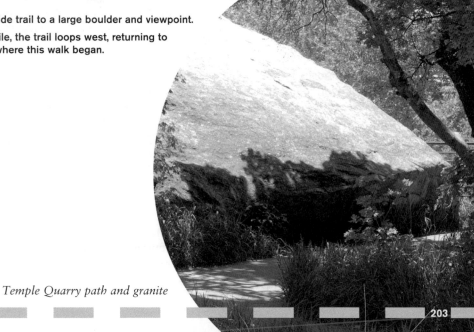

Temple Quarry path and granite

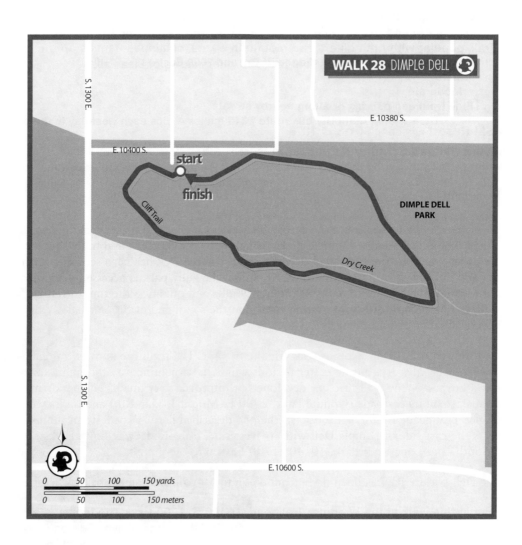

S. 1300 E.

E. 10380 S.

E. 10400 S.

start

finish

Cliff Trail

DIMPLE DELL
PARK

Dry Creek

S. 1300 E.

E. 10600 S.

0   50   100   150 yards

0   50   100   150 meters

28 DIMPLE DELL: a Sandy walk in Sandy

BOUNDARIES: **1300 East, 10400 South, Edgecliff Dr., and 2000 East**
DISTANCE: **1 mile**
DIFFICULTY: **Moderate**
PARKING: **Free trailhead parking or along nearby streets**
PUBLIC TRANSIT: **Utah Transit Authority bus route #313 makes 4 trips each weekday in the area.**

Sandy is a vibrant southern suburb some 14 miles south of downtown Salt Lake City. Here, it is easy to get swallowed by the sprawling community's subdivisions, retail areas, and schools. But running along a generally east-west course through sandy-hilled Sandy is 644-acre Dimple Dell Nature Park.

Smack in the middle of suburbia, the deeply incised gulch is a wild place, generally speaking, albeit one intermittently dammed by crossing highways, its creek and trails squeezed into giant culverts. A slice of nature in an urban setting, Dimple Dell has been set aside for hiking, biking, and horseback riding on unimproved paths. The gully park is accessed via a dozen different trailheads, leading to paths of different kinds and qualities: the rim, the cliff, the bottomland. As such, it offers interesting routes on the south end of the Salt Lake Valley for walkers of all abilities and interests.

But be forewarned: This is also not your usual city park. The trails are above or along a creek bed, which is usually dry, but in wetter periods winds its serpentine way through a tangle of trees and bushes. Many trails are not developed or improved very much. The park's main two trailheads are on its east side (Granite Park, 2900 E. Mount Jordan Rd.) and on its west side (Wrangler Trailhead, 10400 S. 1300 East, the one described here). A pedestrian tunnel also connects the east side of Dimple Dell with its west side, bringing Dewey Bluth Park, 170 E. 9800 South, and Lone Peak Park, 10140 S. 700 East, into the mix.

Dimple Dell Nature Park is open daily from dawn to 10 p.m. Dogs must be on a leash.

● **Begin this walk at the Wrangler Trailhead, 10400 S. 1300 East. The trailhead and parking lot are off 1300 East, southwest of a 24-Hour Fitness gym. The parking lot includes restrooms and picnic pavilions. Head south from the parking lot to a dirt**

Back Story

How did Sandy, Utah's fourth-largest city, get its name? The answer may never be known for certain.

Historians say it may have been named for Alexander "Sandy" Kinghorn, a legendary sandy-bearded, red-haired railroad engineer who hauled cargo and people to the south end of the Salt Lake Valley beginning in 1871. But then again there is the nature of Sandy's underpinning: lumpy, sandy, gullied delta patterns that remind us that the Salt Lake Valley was once swamped by ancient Lake Bonneville, an Ice Age great lake that drained and evaporated thousands of years ago. Pioneer leader Brigham Young himself is said to have given the area its name. As the anecdote goes, he visited, taking one of the first trains serving the area, and said: "Sand! Sand! Everywhere sand! We'll call this place Sandy."

The book *Utah Place Names,* by John W. Van Cott, mentions the "sand bench" on which the community sits. He notes the tale of "Sandy" Kinghorn only in passing, as an alternate claim.

An early newspaper reference to the area's name is a mention of "Sandy station," in the September 13, 1871, issue of the *Deseret News,* where it is described as "the nearest point to Little Cottonwood kanyon (sic)." Historians say Sandy seems to have been first settled in 1871 and had its own post office by 1872.

After walking through the Dimple Dell Nature Park, where loose, sandy paths crisscross the terrain, you might be inclined to agree with the most obvious theory: Sandy is Sandy because of sand.

trail. Take the trailhead's left fork to follow Cliff Trail east for some 300 yards. It skirts the backyard of homes along Edgecliff Dr.

● Turn right to walk down an eroded and steep sandy trail that goes south, amid sagebrush and trees. It is evident that Dimple Dell is heavily used by the valley's equestrians: Horse manure is usually evident along the trail, and you may run into people and horses at the trailhead or along the route. At the bottom of the gully, about 0.3 mile from the trailhead, turn left to walk east. You may have to cross a two-foot-wide shallow section of water here.

- Continue walking east among the groves. There are many dead trees in this area. The bottom of the hollow reduces most of the urban noise generated above. Note that there are myriad trails in the hollow. At 0.5 mile, cross another section of shallow streambed. The sandy bottom lessens the impact of mud on shoes, but they will probably get wet. Only occasional glimpses of houses on the rim above will remind you of civilization.

- Turn left and take the next path north out of the hollow. The uphill climb is quite steep and sandy, as you angle northwest. It should get your heart pumping. At about 0.6 mile, the trail connects with the same path by which you entered the gully.

- Return to Cliff Trail, turn left and walk west, returning to the parking lot and this walk's beginning. This is a simple introduction to Dimple Dell's paths, and it is obvious that longer rambles are possible. If you so desire, you can continue farther east or west in Dimple Dell, but keep track of your position and time; it is a bit of a maze.

route summary

1. Begin this walk at the Wrangler Trailhead, 10400 S. 1300 East. Walk south to the trailhead and turn left (east) to walk along Cliff Trail.

2. Turn right and walk down a steep sandy trail that drops south into the bottom of the gully.

3. At the bottom, turn left to walk east. Depending on the season, you may have to cross a shallow stream several times.

4. After the second stream crossing and at just 0.5 mile out, turn left and walk uphill to the north. Halfway to the rim, fork northwest.

5. Reach Cliff Trail and intersect where you walked down into the gully. Turn left and walk west back to the parking lot and this walk's beginning.

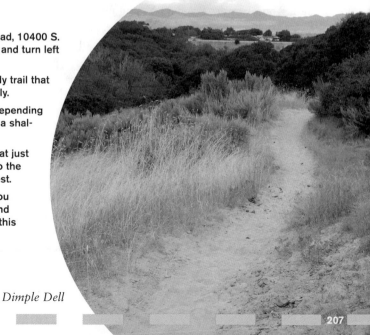

Dimple Dell

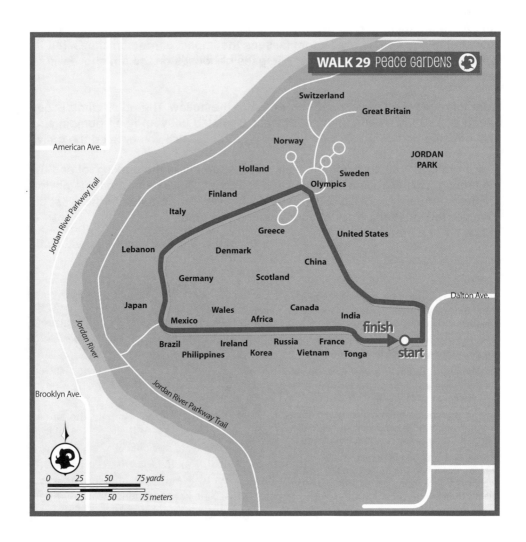

WALK 29 Peace Gardens

Switzerland

Great Britain

Norway

American Ave.

Holland

JORDAN PARK

Sweden

Olympics

Finland

Italy

Greece

United States

Lebanon

Denmark

China

Germany

Scotland

Japan

Wales

Canada

Mexico

Africa

India

Brazil

Ireland

Russia

France

Philippines

Korea

Vietnam

Tonga

finish

start

Dalton Ave.

Jordan River Parkway Trail

Jordan River

Brooklyn Ave.

Jordan River Parkway Trail

| 0 | 25 | 50 | 75 yards |
| 0 | 25 | 50 | 75 meters |

29 THe Peace Gardens: earTH's Nations United

BOUNDARIES: **Northwest section of Jordan Park, 1060 S. 900 West**
DISTANCE: **1 mile**
DIFFICULTY: **Easy**
PARKING: **Free parking inside Jordan Park**
PUBLIC TRANSIT: **Utah Transit Authority bus route #227 travels along 900 West.**

Always wanted to see the world? Switzerland's Matterhorn, perhaps? Or a meditative pathway in Japan? On Salt Lake City's west side—one of the community's more diverse neighborhoods in reality—that concept is miniaturized and compactly presented in Jordan Park's International Peace Gardens. Although in existence for more than six decades and undergoing intermittent changes and additions, the gardens are not particularly well known. "You'd be surprised at how many people don't know about the gardens—we're one of the city's best little secrets," a senior florist told a Salt Lake newspaper a few years ago. Listed in guidebooks, the gardens in summer may host more tourists than locals.

In part that is due to the overall neighborhood's rugged reputation (a point to keep in mind). However, the Peace Gardens, in the northwest corner of Jordan Park, on a curve of the Jordan River, are definitely a bright spot, one worth visiting and strolling. The gardens salute 26 nations, or three times that many if you count those represented in the park's Olympic Peace Pole Circle. Sidewalks, flowers, lawns, mature trees, and hedges border and link familiar architectural styles and international icons, such as the little Matterhorn and Denmark's *Little Mermaid*.

Credit for the Peace Gardens concept goes to Mrs. Otto (Ruey) Wiesley and the Salt Lake Council of Women. Ruey Wiesley proposed the concept in 1939, and by early 1941 she had the support of the Salt Lake City government. However war, not peace, was in the process of engulfing the planet, as nations chose sides in World War II. It wasn't until 1947 that an American section was completed in Jordan Park, soon followed by a Japanese area, a postwar rapprochement truly emblematic of the park's ideals. Salt Lake residents from many lands took up the idea, and the Peace Gardens were formally dedicated in 1952.

While amity and unity are the hope, several Peace Gardens plaques are missing—some stolen, some in disrepair and in storage. Graffiti speckles and spoils other spots. The lawns and gardens are well tended, though they too have faced budget cuts in recent difficult financial times, newspapers report. Some architectural landscaping could use a bit of tender, loving care and an infusion of dollars. Still, Jordan Park and the International Peace Gardens are well worth a visit. The gardens are relatively safe during the daytime, and of course picnic and playground areas are available in the larger park. Jordan Park's International Peace Gardens are open daily, 7 a.m.–11 p.m. Admission is free. Smoking is not allowed in the park, and dogs must be on a leash.

- Begin this walk in the northwest corner of Jordan Park, which is on the west side of 900 West at 1050 South. Use the northernmost entrance (the north arm of the park's U-shaped Dalton Ave.) and northwest parking areas. Proceed north to an arched gateway that says "International Peace Gardens." These directions will have you following the main sidewalk in a counterclockwise direction. Plaques on the stonework supporting the 1955 entryway's wrought-iron arch summarize the garden's founding and its purpose. Its objective is "to work for peace by fostering international brotherhood among the peoples of the world. These various garden plots, in landscaping, design, planting and architecture, are symbolic of the nations they represent. Situated as they are, side by side, in a friendly grouping, these plots typify the spirit of international amity and understanding." Other plaques beyond the gate honor Mrs. Wiesley and other advocates.

- As the garden's interior loop begins, turn right, walking north. To the right again, in a large grassy area on the east, is the park's section devoted to the host nation, the United States. Plantings spell out "America." Three flagpoles rise in the background, and to the north, requiring a walk across the lawn for a closer look, is a Peace on Earth monument dedicated in 1976—America's bicentennial—expressing "Our hope for the children." The artwork is by prominent Utah sculptor Avard Fairbanks. On the other side of the sidewalk, to the left (west), is a Chinese gate with a red-tiled roof, and then, also on the left, an elegant set of Grecian pillars.

- Next up, as the walk continues north, is a circle festooned with wooden "peace poles." These commemorate the 2002 Winter Olympic Games, hosted by Salt Lake City. The 84 poles stood in the Salt Lake City & County Building's central Washington Square during the competition and festival. Each bears text in support of the "Olympic Truce," calling for solidarity, cooperation, and friendship among nations. Lettering in English, French, and another representative language—Fijian, Spanish, Chinese, Russian, etc.—makes a plea for peace within and between nations. All say: "May peace prevail on Earth."

● Straight ahead, European states predominate. A prominent Swiss section is to the right (north), with a child-sized chalet and the delightful mini Matterhorn, perhaps 30 feet tall. Tucked away to the northeast, somewhat hidden on an offshoot path, is an English garden, rededicated in 2000 with the addition of a bust of Margaret Thatcher, the nation's first woman prime minister. "We hoped the Queen wasn't too offended!" a pair of traveling bloggers observed after a park visit in 2002.

● As the main sidewalk swerves left and to the west, Scandinavia takes center stage. First up, even before the Swiss display, is a discreet Swedish garden, just north of the U.S. section. Norway's updated garden features a raised memorial Bauta stone inscribed with images and runes, a symbol of Norwegian heritage erected in 2008. Across the way, on the walkway's left (south) side, Denmark joins in with a gravel, bowery-covered trail leading to a pool (sometimes disconcertingly empty) with a reduced-size replica of sculptor Edvard Eriksen's *Little Mermaid.* A Scottish area is tucked in to the east, between the Danish and Chinese sections. Nearby to the right (north) is Holland's plot, followed by a fine pine grove established by Finland's advocates. You may note that the Jordan River is swinging around the north and west sides of the Peace Gardens here, with a separate, paved path that connects with the gardens.

● The park walkway next passes a tribute to Italy, on the right, represented

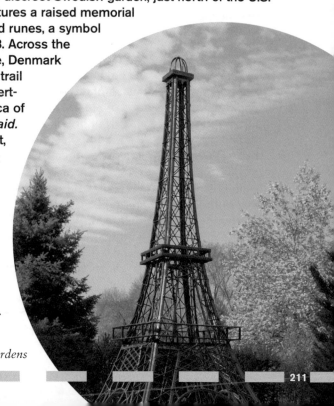

Eiffel Tower replica, International Peace Gardens

by a familiar image of its bootlike peninsula, as well as the Mediterranean isles of Sicily and Sardinia, all on a mosaic-tile sea of cerulean blue. Germany is across the way, on the left. The exhibit features sculpted hedges, memorial park benches, a landscape well, and a castle gate. The accompanying plaque is written entirely in German. Lebanon's small garden is next door.

- On the Peace Gardens' westernmost bend is a pleasing highlight, an exhibit honoring Japan. The garden is graced with a small pagoda, little arched bridges, and a pillar lantern. A 1997 marker mentions Utah's statehood centennial (in 1996), as well as the 50th anniversary of Japanese-American participation in the International Peace Gardens. Nearby is a link to the Jordan River Parkway Trail and a pedestrian bridge to the Jordan River's west side.

- On the sidewalk's left side, toward the route's center, is Mexico's garden, with a massive Toltec-style head as its centerpiece and a round stone replica of a Mayan calendar. Brazil's modest plot is across the path, in the Peace Gardens' southwestern corner, and a Philippine section is just to the east of that.

- As the sidewalk heads east, the Korean Garden, on the path's right (south) side is one of the most extensive of all. The Korean War was raging, of course, as these gardens built up a head of steam, though markers bear dates more recent. Covering a larger area than most, the Korean section features two areas with elaborate, tile-topped stone walls, inscribed poles, and several memorial plaques. One marker notes that a vanished pavilion once stood in the area.

- Continuing east, on the path's right are Russia's garden (with a metallic 1990s map of the federation) and Ireland (with a Celtic cross). On the left, in the park's center, are tributes to Wales (with a graceful harp monument); the nations of Africa, collectively; African-Americans (a hewn stone marker); and Canada (a grove and rock garden).

- Vietnam is next on the right, distinguished by a red gate and two regal white lions, followed by France, with landscaping that features—what else—a five-foot replica of the Eiffel Tower. India's garden is on the inside left as you near the conclusion to the Peace Gardens loop, presenting a bust of Mahatma Gandhi and a raised plaque with a preaching Buddha. A Tongan section, one marker noting the island nation's independence day, is on the right as you return to this walk's beginning.

POINT OF INTEREST

International Peace Gardens at Jordan Park internationalpeacegardens.org,
1060 S. 900 West, 801-938-5326

ROUTE SUMMARY

1. Begin this walk in the northwest corner of Jordan Park. Enter on U-shaped Dalton Ave.'s northern arm, off 900 West at about 1060 South, and continue west to park if you are in a vehicle.

2. Walk north to and through the International Peace Gardens' arched entryway.

3. Follow the central loop counterclockwise; leave the path and cross lawns if you wish to visit some displays and monuments.

4. The loop proceeds north, then west, and curves briefly south before returning east to the start. The route is less than a mile, with several possible temporary offshoots into specific national garden sections.

CONNECTING THE WALKS

Connect with Walk 30, Jordan River Parkway, at the west end of the International Peace Gardens, where the routes intersect, or at other points in the gardens and in Jordan Park.

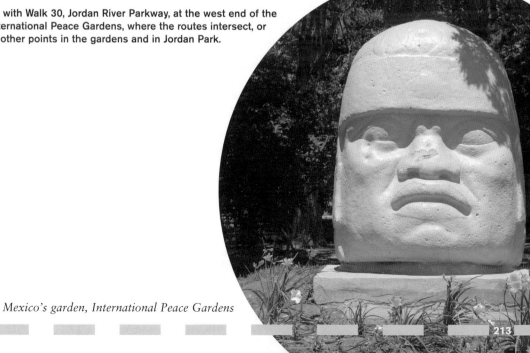

Mexico's garden, International Peace Gardens

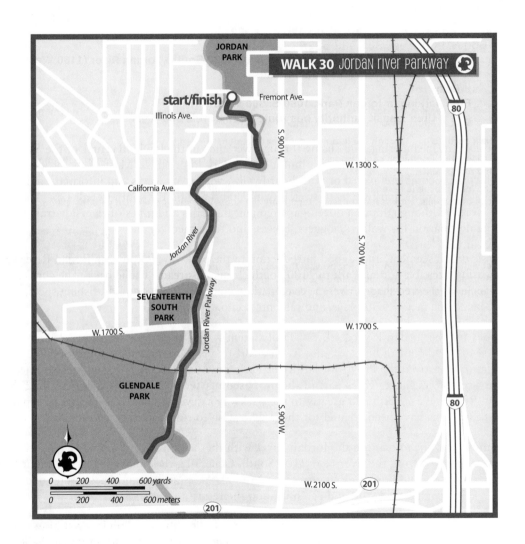

JORDAN PARK

WALK 30 Jordan River Parkway

start/finish

Fremont Ave.

Illinois Ave.

S. 900 W.

W. 1300 S.

California Ave.

Jordan River

S. 700 W.

SEVENTEENTH SOUTH PARK

Jordan River Parkway

W. 1700 S.

W. 1700 S.

GLENDALE PARK

S. 900 W.

0   200   400   600 yards
0   200   400   600 meters

W. 2100 S.

201

80

80

201

30 Jordan River Parkway: a river runs through it

BOUNDARIES: 1000 South, 900 West, California Ave. (1330 South), Jordan River (1100 West)
DISTANCE: 2 miles, with options for 3 and 4 miles
DIFFICULTY: Easy
PARKING: Free parking in Jordan Park, 1060 S. 900 West
PUBLIC TRANSIT: Utah Transit Authority bus route #227 travels 900 West

Generally flat, meandering, and slicing through wetlands in the lowland center of the Salt Lake Valley, the Jordan River Parkway is a multidecade work in progress. Most of the proposed 40-mile trail is complete: paved or with boardwalks, with river access and informational signs. Eventually the public parkway is to stretch from Utah Lake on the south to Salt Lake City's 1000 North. Although about a dozen gaps remain, the miles and miles of riverside trail are a favorite destination for walkers, joggers, bikers, and fishermen.

A classic urban segment, and a good introduction to the parkway, follows the Jordan River south from easily accessible Jordan Park to 2100 South: 1 mile upstream, 1 mile back. The curvaceous route includes the tree-shaded river, a paved path, picnic parks, playgrounds, fishing spots, canoe-launching facilities, displays, and safe intersection crossings.

The idea for the Jordan River Parkway Trail system was born 40 years ago, in 1971, as a method of flood control but soon also as an effort to clean up midvalley pollution. The Utah Legislature approved the Provo-Jordan River Parkway Authority in 1973, while also rejecting two reservoirs suggested as part of the proposed master plan. Individual cities along the Jordan River have contributed greatly to the parkway's development. In some areas, separate equestrian paths have been created for those who wish to ride horses along the river.

It is important not to confuse the Jordan River with the Jordan River Surplus Canal, which diverts northwest from the river near 2100 South. Generally, the canal runs in a straight line, and it lacks trees and bushes along its course. And as this is an out-and-back route, one can always skip a sightseeing stop and catch it upon the return.

● **Begin on the west side of Jordan Park, after entering the park on its east side via Dalton Ave., at 1050 S. 900 West, where sidewalks connect to the parkway. Walk** south. In about a third of a mile you will reach Bend-in-the-River, a green-space mini-park created by volunteers, community members, and elementary school students. One highlight of the two-acre site is the Urban Tree House, a covered gathering place. And ahoy, mateys! Nearby is a play spot that looks much like a sailing ship, with boardwalk planks and mastlike poles ideal for exercising the imaginations of young Jack Sparrows, Elizabeth Swanns, and Will Turners. Nature displays dot the wayside, offering tidbits about the Jordan: "Do fish live in the river? Answer: Yes! Utah chub, common carp, catfish, and rainbow trout all call the Jordan River 'home.'"

- Continuing south, cross a bridge a half mile from the start, and then note a canoe-launching area at 0.7 mile. 1300 South is generally not a busy road. Then, a large field opens up—covered not with grass but with a natural riverside habitat. Off to the side and worth a diversion is The River of Words Peace Labyrinth, about 100 feet to the right of the main trail via a short dirt path. Colorful tile artwork patterns represent the Jordan River, Salt Lake area and Utah scenery, flowers, fish, a butterfly, meditative mandalas, and a host of other things.

- At 1 mile, you reach California Ave. (1330 South). A busy street, this is the turnaround point if you would like a simple 2-mile stroll. Reverse course and return to Jordan Park along the same path. On either side of the parkway is a mix of old and new homes.

- If you wish a longer walk, push the crosswalk button to safely ford California Ave. and continue southward. This is more of an industrial-park area, lined with businesses and parking lots full of cars and trucks.

- Continuing south, you will reach the intersection of 1700 South, 1.5 miles from the route's start. Turn around and return to Jordan Park if you wish a 3-mile trek. Unfortunately defaced, an informational sign indicates that this section of the parkway was designated part of the Utah Millennium Trail in 2000.

- Once again, if you want to continue your walk, push the automated crosswalk button to get across the busy highway. You will also soon cross over an active railroad track that lacks an electronic crossing apparatus. Although trains aren't roaring along this east-west side track, listen and look both ways before proceeding over the rails. Nearby you may note, to the west, the soaring water slides and playful screams of Seven Peaks Waterpark (formerly Raging Waters).

● At 2 full miles from the start, the path veers southwest, where you can clearly see the diverging Jordan River Surplus Canal. Stop, reverse course and turn around here, retracing the parkway path to the start to complete a 4-mile walk. (The trail continues farther south, swinging right and west to a bridge, then passing under the 2100 South Freeway.)

POINTS OF INTEREST (START TO FINISH)

International Peace Gardens at Jordan Park internationalpeacegardens.org,
1060 S. 900 West, 801-938-5326

Seven Peaks Waterpark ragingwatersutah.com, 1200 W. 1700 South, 801-972-3300

ROUTE SUMMARY

1. Begin this walk on the west side of Jordan Park, accessed via the park's east side and Dalton Ave., at 1050 S. 900 West.
2. Walk south on the defined, paved Jordan River Parkway Trail, on the east side of the Jordan River.
3. California Ave. (1330 South) is the 1-mile mark; for a 2-mile round-trip stroll, turn around and return to Jordan Park.
4. If you want a longer walk, push the automated signal switch and cross California Ave., when the green pedestrian signal is indicated, to pick up the trail.
5. Continue south to the intersection at 1700 South; this is 1.5 miles from the walk's start. Once again, push the crosswalk button to get across the highway to access the continuing trail. Or turn around and return to Jordan Park for a 3-mile walk.
6. Watch for, and cross safely, an occasionally used railroad crossing just beyond 1700 South.
7. Near 2100 South, a busy freeway, you will have walked 2 miles. Nearby is the Jordan River Surplus Canal. This is the turnaround point for a 4-mile walk. Retrace the trail to Jordan Park to complete the walk.

CONNECTING THE WALKS

Connect with Walk 29, The Peace Gardens, in the northwest corner of Jordan Park, where this route also begins.

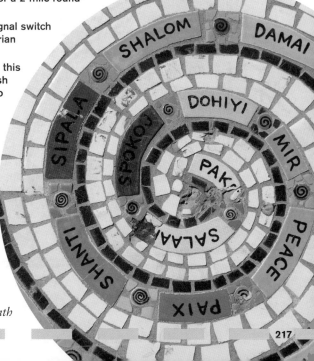

Peace Labyrinth

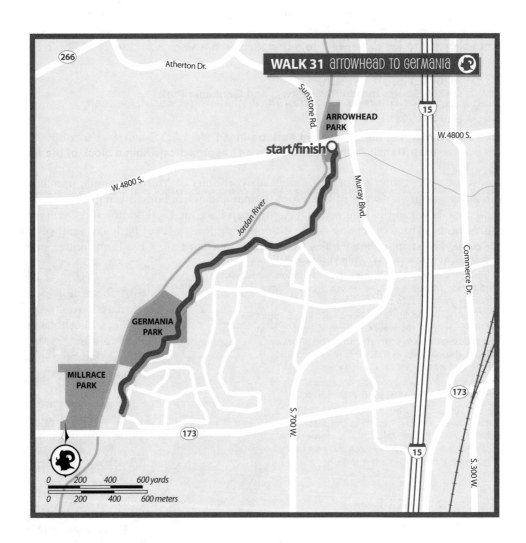

266

Atherton Dr.

Sunstone Rd.

15

W. 4800 S.

ARROWHEAD PARK

start/finish

W. 4800 S.

Murray Blvd.

Jordan River

Commerce Dr.

GERMANIA PARK

MILLRACE PARK

S. 700 W.

173

173

S. 300 W.

15

0   200   400   600 yards

0   200   400   600 meters

31 arrowHeaD TO Germania: JorDan river's riBBON OF LIFE

BOUNDARIES: 4800 South, Jordan River Pkwy., and Germania Park
DISTANCE: 3 miles
DIFFICULTY: Easy
PARKING: Free parking at the Arrowhead Park trailhead
PUBLIC TRANSIT: Utah Transit Authority bus route #47 approaches within a block of the trailhead.

In almost the exact center of the Salt Lake Valley, the city of Murray's 5-mile stretch of the Jordan River is truly a ribbon of life. Flora, fauna, and active human beings flourish in the wetland zone between the community's Arrowhead Park (at 4800 South) and Germania Park (at 5400 South). This key section of the 40-mile-long Jordan River Parkway Trail system is a nature park. The strip, about 5 miles from downtown Salt Lake City, is a prime example of what has been done to improve the multiuse parkway.

This walk's starting point, a little picnic ground and trailhead called Arrowhead Park, gets its name from Native American weaponry discovered in the area. The Jordan River and tributary creeks provided seasonal camping and hunting for tribes such as the Piute, Shoshone, and Ute well before Anglo-Saxon and other settlers arrived, and they continued to use the area as late as 1910, a historical marker notes. From their camps they traded tanned skins and meats for other supplies and food.

Midway between the two bracketing parks is the Nature Center of Murray. Dedicated in 1999, the open-air encounter with Mother Nature includes overlooks above the Jordan River wetlands and a larger viewpoint deck above an amphitheater and marsh. It is not uncommon to see local preschoolers and elementary-school students walking the paths and getting first-hand exposure to nature in what is otherwise the suburban Salt Lake area. Besides the foot-path, an equestrian trail follows the Jordan River here.

All in all, the Arrowhead-to-Germania trail offers an excellent example of what the best jaunts along the Jordan River Parkway Trail can be like in Salt Lake County and northern Utah County. (For more about the Jordan River Parkway, see Walk 30.)

- Begin this walk at Murray's Arrowhead Park, 593 W. 4800 South, on the Jordan River Parkway Trail. Walk south along the river's east side on a paved trail and boardwalk. The path often has a center yellow line to divide north-south traffic. However, beware speeding cyclists along this trail, especially during the first 0.2 mile, where an extra-narrow boardwalk can funnel pedestrians and bikes into closer proximity.

- After crossing a small bridge and proceeding along the boardwalk section, the trail opens up to a wider, two-lane configuration, complete with those yellow divider dashes. At 0.4 mile, wetlands begin in earnest. Three separate side trails offer close-up excursions among the reeds and ponds beside the Jordan River. Birders have espied scores of species along here, from common mallards, redhead and overwintering green-teal ducks to great blue herons, American white pelicans, bald eagles, and a variety of hummingbirds.

- Along the way, note signs presenting mini-histories of life beside the Jordan River. One such placard points out that the pioneer Snarr family settled this area, originally called the Big Cottonwood Precinct. James Thomas Snarr's clan homesteaded a 30-acre farm and a 20-acre pasture, and descendants grew garden vegetables and raised milk cows to provide products for a store the family owned in Salt Lake City. The primary crop, however, was sugar beets, a prominent industry in the Intermountain West at one time. The Snarrs remain prominent in local business and Murray politics to this day.

- Another trail access point is near the halfway point of this trail segment, at Lucky Clover Lane (5040 South) and Morning Dew Dr. (770 West). There is a small parking lot near the Nature Center of Murray. The center, created with financial assistance from the Kennecott Utah Copper Corp., which operates the huge open-pit mine visible in the Oquirrh Mountains to the west, is managed by the Murray School District. It serves as a natural biology and conservation classroom for elementary school students. Interpretive signs illuminate all passersby who pause, offering a bird's-eye view map of the Salt Lake Valley and the Jordan River, an explanation of wetlands' roles, and a description of the area's diverse bird life.

- Walk up a slight hill near the nature center area. Be sure to take the 50-yard side path to the right that leads to an impressive overlook of the Jordan River wetlands. Small green nature-trail markers point out flowers and foliage such as coyote willow, blanketflowers, wild blue flax, and Shasta daisies.

- Continue walking south. At 0.7 mile, the dirt equestrian trail is visible to the right; many walkers and mountain bikers choose to use it instead of the paved trail.

- At 0.9 mile, a side path heads west across a bridge over the Jordan River. It leads to another path and access to neighborhoods on the river's west side. The bridge offers excellent views of both the river and its central place in the Salt Lake Valley. The Oquirrh Mountains loom to the west, and the Wasatch Mountains rise sharply to the east.

- At 1.2 miles, the path splits in two as it reaches the north edge of Germania Park. Germania is larger than Arrowhead Park, with a large picnic pavilion, a playground, barbecue pits, a basketball court, and multipurpose sports fields. Loop this area and head north, returning to Arrowhead Park, for a 3-mile round-trip Jordan River Parkway walk.

POINTS OF INTEREST (START TO FINISH)

Arrowhead Park murray.utah.gov, 593 W. 4800 South

Kennecott Nature Center of Murray
murrayschools.org/kennecott-nature-center,
5044 S. Lucky Clover Lane

Germania Park murray.utah.gov, 5243 S.
Murray Parkway Ave.

ROUTE SUMMARY

1. Begin at the Arrowhead Park/Jordan River Parkway trailhead, 593 W. 4800 South.
2. Walk south along the east side of the Jordan River, on the paved trail and boardwalk.
3. Continue 1.5 miles to Germania Park.
4. Turn around and return along the same path to Arrowhead Park.

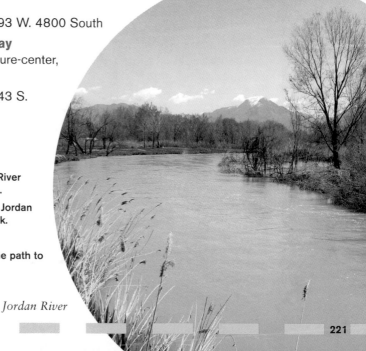

Jordan River

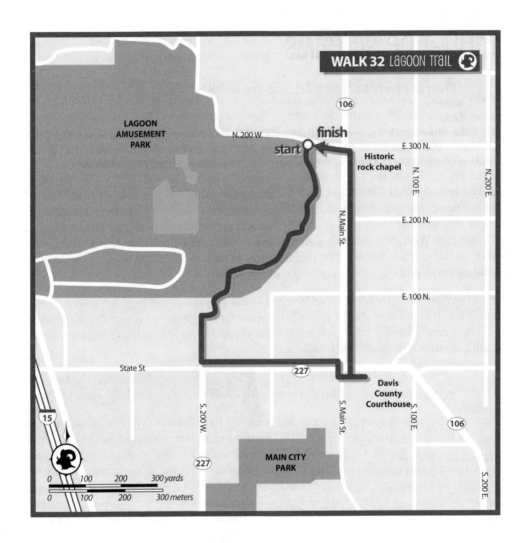

WALK 32 Lagoon Trail

LAGOON AMUSEMENT PARK

106

N. 200 W.

finish
start

E. 300 N.

Historic rock chapel

N. 100 E.

N. 200 E.

E. 200 N.

N. Main St.

E. 100 N.

State St

227

Davis County Courthouse

S. 200 W.

S. Main St.

S. 100 E.

106

227

MAIN CITY PARK

S. 200 E.

15

0   100   200   300 yards
0   100   200   300 meters

32 Lagoon Trail: Village Dreams, Thrill-ride Screams

BOUNDARIES: **Main St., State St., 200 West, and 300 North**
DISTANCE: **1 mile**
DIFFICULTY: **Easy**
PARKING: **Free street parking or in nearby church lot; avoid areas where signs restrict parking.**
PUBLIC TRANSIT: **Utah Transit Authority bus route #470 serves Farmington's Main St.; a summer shuttle bus connects Lagoon theme park and the Davis County Courthouse.**

Charming Farmington, 16 miles north of Salt Lake City via I-15, is a magnet for locals and visitors alike. That can be attributed partly to the picture-book appeal of its tree-canopied streets, but largely it is because this small town is home to Lagoon theme park, the Dramamine capital of the Mountain West. Stuffed with roller coasters old-fashioned and new, swimming facilities, and other attractions for fun-seekers, the amusement park is the oldest west of the Mississippi River and indeed one of the most venerable in the world.

A visit to Lagoon will give any walker's legs a good workout (and perhaps a few wobbles), but there's no denying that theme parks are expensive. Lagoon "passports" for two adults, plus parking, can easily set you back $100. The thrills, in addition to the more peaceful appeal of Lagoon's Pioneer Village, may well be worth it.

But a free stroll just beyond the screams is possible along the park's fringes, on the Lagoon Trail, with a loop through historic downtown Farmington. A village walk might prove just the ticket.

Farmington, a suburban county seat nestled between the Wasatch Mountains and the eastern shore of the Great Salt Lake, was settled soon after pioneers arrived in Utah in 1847 and originally was called North Cottonwood. The community's many traditional rock-façade buildings, from residences to churches and public structures, are an enduring reminder of that heritage. Incorporated in 1892, Farmington, today with a population of about 14,000, has also been known as Utah's City of Roses. Indeed, blooming roses continue, in season, to sprinkle pastel color throughout the community. Farmington's fragrant gardens, tree-lined streets, and general lack of urban commercialization add to a setting that offers an opportunity for a refreshing amble through the hometown you might never have had.

BaCK STOrY

Utah's Lagoon amusement park actually got its start as Lake Park Resort on the shores of the Great Salt Lake on July 15, 1886. It received its current name in 1896, when it moved inland, next to a small lake, or "lagoon," and adjacent to magnate–park owner Simon Bamberger's rail line. Today the park boasts 45 rides, including world-class roller coasters; a water park dubbed Lagoon-A-Beach; entertainment venues; and historic Pioneer Village.

Lagoon also offers an unusual perk most amusement parks do not: it allows outside food to be taken inside its gates and boasts more than a dozen picnic areas. Often a site of family reunions and church gatherings, it is Utah's fourth most visited tourist attraction, with more than 1.2 million visitors annually.

Besides the park's thrill rides and entertainment offerings, Lagoon is home to Pioneer Village, a bonus that includes 42 authentic 19th-century Utah buildings spread over about 15 acres. Most of the preserved structures were first brought together in Salt Lake City, until the village was moved lock, stock, and barrel in 1976 to Lagoon's east side. The park's Rattlesnake Rapids and Log Flume rides add to zone's Old West flavor.

Pioneer Village includes a rock chapel, originally raised in 1853 as a fort in Coalville, Utah. Among the village's other structures are a one-room schoolhouse, a two-story log house, a smokehouse, a millinery, a clock shop, a tool museum, a music hall, a museum, and, of course, a town hall.

The Pioneer Village is like "stepping into yesteryear," Peter Freed, Lagoon's president, said when the village premiered. "It brings to life the way people lived during the first 100 years of Utah's existence."

● Begin your Farmington walk at Main St. and 300 North. Park curbside on 300 North by the LDS Church or in its lot, on the intersection's southeast corner, though there is space to park one or two vehicles nearer the entry to the Lagoon Trail, which actually begins about a quarter-block west, across Main St.

● The Lagoon Trail's entrance, about 200 feet west of the intersection, on the south side of 300 North, is marked by a small covered bridge. From the entry, walk south on a wide asphalt trail. Greenhouses sit on the path's east side (300 North's south side), helping furnish Lagoon's immaculate flower gardens. To the west (right), you can catch glimpses of the theme park's Rattlesnake Rapids water ride, an artificial river that carries up to eight passengers on huge tubes through Old West–themed splashes and thrills. The trail swings back and forth, though be wary of bicycle riders, who may speed along the path.

- As you stroll south amid trees and beyond old farm outbuildings, benches offer opportunities to sit and rest. If Lagoon is open at the time, you will hear various theme-park sounds—clangs, shrieks, laughter, and such. After only about 250 yards of walking, you will pass by a section of Lagoon's zoo, beyond the trail's western fence. Yes, this theme park has an extensive zoo, including bears, lions, birds, and camels. Along the Lagoon Trail you are most likely to see deer, elk, and a small herd of bison (or buffalo), including lively light-brown calves. As signs advise, don't try to feed these animals, and keep your distance: only a tall chain-link fence separates these huge animals from people on the trail.

- Continuing southwest, the pathway's country feel is bolstered by small horse pastures on its east side. As you wind past Lagoon's electrical power stations, the Lagoon Trail path itself ends after only 0.3 mile, as it intersects a longer trail (which connects to the 3.7-mile Farmington Creek Trail and the freeway's frontage road jogging path). Walk another 0.1 mile south to the dead end of 200 West (also known as Walker Lane).

- Walk south on the right, or western, side of this residential street to State St. Near the intersection's northwest corner are historical markers. One notes that this is the Clark Lane National Historic District, settled by the descendants of pioneer Ezra Thompson Clark. Another tells the story of the Bamberger Railroad station that also stood nearby, with rails running north and south along 200 West. The interurban line served passengers between Salt Lake City and Ogden from the 1890s to the 1950s, with Farmington halfway between the two metropolises. Lagoon itself was established by entrepreneur Simon Bamberger as an added attraction and destination for his customers.

- From the intersection of 200 West and State St., walk east two blocks to Farmington's Main St. Historic homes line the thoroughfare, some dating back to the 1850s and 1860s.

- At the signaled intersection of Main and State Sts., turn right to cross to the south side of State St. Then, turn left and cross Main St., walking east. Near the corner stands an eye-catching red-, white-, and blue-painted bison statue, part of a community art project. The large edifice on your right is Farmington's Davis County Courthouse. Built in classical Roman style with six front pillars, it opened in 1932. A sidewalk map illustrates the county's size and placement beside the Great Salt Lake. To the east, at 88 E. State St., is the rock-faced VanFleet Hotel, built in the 1850s and now serving as dental offices. (A service station with a convenience store is just around the curving corner to the northeast.)

- After taking in Farmington's historic center, turn around and walk west, returning to the junction of Main and State Sts.

- At the intersection's southeast corner, turn right to cross with the signal to the north side of State St., and continue walking north on Farmington's leafy, sycamore-lined Main St. (A barbershop and a gift shop called Just a Bed of Roses are a few doors up the north side of State St.)

- Walking north on Main you will pass Aunt Addy's, an antiques store, as well as many homes and the original redbrick Farmington City Hall, complete with a replica Civil War cannon out front. Today it is Farmington's historical museum, with limited hours. At 272 N. Main St. is the Mormon rock meetinghouse. As a historical marker notes, the chapel's core was built in 1862–63, though the structure has been enlarged and remodeled twice in the century and a half since. It was also the site of the first-ever Mormon Primary meeting in 1878, a physical and spiritual program that today serves young children throughout the LDS Church.

- This is where this walk began, at 300 North and Main St. If you parked a vehicle nearer the Lagoon Trail entrance, it is across Main St. to the west on 300 North.

POINTS OF INTEREST (START TO FINISH)

Lagoon Theme Park lagoonpark.com, 375 Lagoon Dr., 801-451-8000

Lagoon RV Park and Campground lagoonpark.com/parkinfo/camping, 375 N. Lagoon Dr., 801-451-8100

Just a Bed of Roses justabedofroses.blogspot.com, 15 E. State St., 801-628-0890

Aunt Addy's Country Home 58 N. Main St., 801-451-6400

route summary

1. Begin this walk about 200 feet west of the intersection of Farmington's Main St. and 300 North. The Lagoon Trail covered-bridge entrance is on the south side of 300 North.

2. Walk south on the wide asphalt trail. The path winds back and forth, with rural property on the left (east) and the Lagoon amusement park on the right (west). Watch for bicycle traffic using the same route.

3. After walking 0.3 mile you will reach another north-south path; proceed south to the dead end of residential 200 West (also known as Walker Lane), and the end of the formal Lagoon Trail. Walk south on the right (west) side of the road to State St., where there are historical markers.

4. Walk east on State St. two blocks to Main St.

5. Turn right, crossing at the signal to the south side of State St.; then, again at the signal, turn left to cross Main St., walking east.

6. The Davis County Courthouse is on the intersection's southeast corner. Look it over and then turn around and walk west to return to the intersection of Main and State Sts.

7. Turn right and cross to the north side of State St., continuing north along Main St. for three blocks.

8. Just before the junction of Main St. and 300 North, at 272 N. Main St., is Farmington's historic rock chapel. You may have parked a vehicle here on 300 North; if you parked nearer the beginning of the Lagoon Trail, it is across Main St. to the west on 300 North.

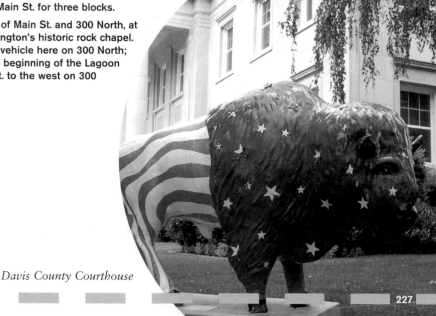

Davis County Courthouse

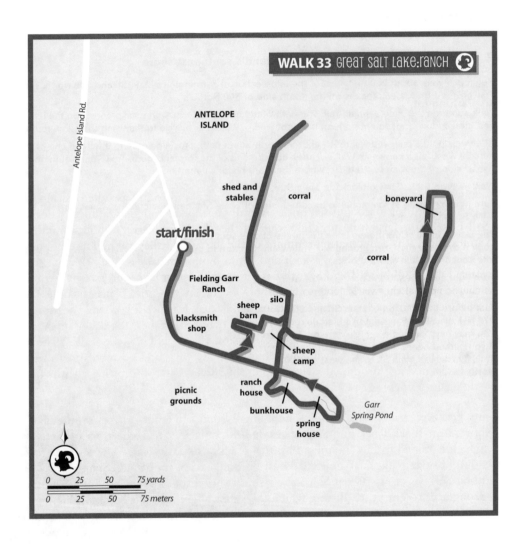

ANTELOPE ISLAND

Antelope Island Rd.

shed and stables

corral

boneyard

start/finish

corral

Fielding Garr Ranch

silo

blacksmith shop

sheep barn

sheep camp

picnic grounds

ranch house

bunkhouse

spring house

Garr Spring Pond

0   25   50   75 yards

0   25   50   75 meters

33 Great Salt Lake: Ranch

BOUNDARIES: Fielding Garr Ranch, Antelope Island's southeast shore
DISTANCE: 1 mile
DIFFICULTY: Easy
PARKING: Parking lot
PUBLIC TRANSIT: None available

The vast lake mere miles west and north of Salt Lake City is not your usual watery pleasure zone.

Utah's capital is really, of course, "Great Salt Lake City," and so it was called during its first few decades, named for an inland sea both generally dismissed and geographically dominant. Great Salt Lake is the largest natural lake west of the Mississippi River. About 75 miles long and 35 miles wide, it is a fluctuating remnant of the Ice Age's valley-filling Lake Bonneville. Today's lake puddles west of the Wasatch and Uinta mountain ranges, the principal sources of its water. Like the Biblical Dead Sea, this is a terminal desert lake—no rivers flow out of it toward the oceans of the world. Evaporation, however, leaves behind concentrations of salt and other minerals, much desired by extraction industries. It is not a lakeside vacation draw in the usual sense, surrounded by lodges and family cabins. At times, the decay of shore vegetation, where freshwater meets salt water, is pungent. Locals call it "lake stink." The lake is much saltier than the ocean, which causes buoyancy. Resorts and postcards in an earlier, more lake-fascinated age promoted swimming in the saline water, promising visitors they would "float like a cork!"

There are, however, true pleasures to be had. Small boats sail from harbors on the lake's south shore, near Black Rock and Saltair beside I-80, and on the northern tip of Antelope Island, which is joined to the "mainland" north of Salt Lake City via a fine causeway. The artificial land bridge makes a 7-mile east-west beeline, except for a single major elbowlike kink. Public beaches are on Great Salt Lake's south shore, though they fell into neglect during a long drought in recent years, during which the lake's shoreline receded, exposing its muddy bed. The best beaches—for those who wish to dip toes in the water or walk the shores on light, rounded oolitic sand—are on the northern and northwestern shores of Antelope Island. At intervals the isle has been considered a potential national park. The state of Utah acquired

2,000 acres on the north in 1969 for a small park, and then in 1981 purchased all 28,022 acres to create Antelope Island State Park. For many visitors, Antelope Island is the best way to experience the Great Salt Lake.

For much of its history, though, Antelope Island—the largest of the lake's nine—was a huge ranch. Because of a mountainous spine and island shoreline, few fences were needed. From the earliest pioneer days, horses, cattle, pigs, and eventually bison—popularly known as buffalo—were brought here to graze its grasses, along with native deer, bighorn sheep, and pronghorn antelope. Today it is a bison refuge, with between 500 and 700 of the great shaggy beasts, which faced extinction just a century ago. Birds abound, too: The islands and less-salty shoreline wetlands are key western segments of North America's migratory Central Flyway. American avocets, long-billed curlews, ferruginous hawks, California gulls, a variety of duck species, and bald eagles, among scores of other winged creatures, draw birders from around the world. The Great Salt Lake is pretty lively for a dead sea.

Simple beach strolls are possible along Bridger and Whiterock Bays, complicated at times by flurries of nonbiting brine flies and more annoying tiny biting flies, known as no-see-ums. The shore can also be striped with dark, drying ribbons of brine shrimp, the lake's dominant life-form—it has no fish. Buffalo Point offers a short hillside hike on the island's northwest edge. Frary Peak, the 6,596-foot summit, is a more taxing 7-mile round-trip hike with a great reward: a high island view, circled by water, mountains, and sky. There are several other hiking routes, as well.

We're recommending a simpler walk at historic Fielding Garr Ranch, one suitable for the whole family. Garr was the first to settle here, in 1848. From the ranch compound, modern Salt Lake City's skyline can be seen flickering like a mirage only a few miles distant, below high mountain peaks. Antelope Island also has a small visitor center and museum, with a gift shop. Island Buffalo Grill (offering buffalo burgers!) operates seasonally on Bridger Bay.

Access to Antelope Island, about 40 miles north of Salt Lake City, is via Antelope Dr., off exit 332 in Layton. Drive west through Syracuse to the park entrance and causeway. There is a $9 day-use fee per vehicle. The cost is $6 for those cars with a senior age 62 or over, and $3 for cyclists and pedestrians. (Yes, the causeway itself is a biking and walking candidate.) Fielding Garr Ranch is reached via the island's eastern shoreline drive, a left (south) turn at the causeway's end. Access to the park is during daylight hours (the gates close, though there are overnight campgrounds). The visitor center and ranch are open 9 a.m.–6 p.m. in spring and summer, and until 5 in other seasons. The park itself opens at 7 a.m. and closes variably between 6 and 10 p.m., depending upon the season. The east-shore drive to Fielding Garr Ranch presents excellent views of the Wasatch Mountains, the city and suburbs, and what government explorer Howard Stansbury described, in 1850, as "a great and peculiar beauty."

- Walk from the parking lot east, downhill into the Fielding Garr Ranch compound. Just past a large dinner bell, which is on the southeast corner of the blacksmith's shed, turn left and head north. You will see an entrance to an orientation room and museum inside the stone, timber, and corrugated-metal barn. Guides and rangers are in the vicinity. They can help you get started or even lead you on a tour.

- Step inside the little museum, chockablock with informational placards, photographs, tools, a soft bison hide hanging from the rock wall, and skulls of bison, deer, and big-horn sheep. Touching things is quite OK here, says historian-curator Clay Shelley—playful kids even like to put pointy deer antlers, stacked in a corner, on their heads. The museum room and the ranch itself represent more than 160 years and several eras. Beginning in 1848, the island was used for grazing by area's settlers and by The Church of Jesus Christ of Latter-day Saints. Salt Lake City was the only Anglo-American village between Missouri and the West Coast. To help fund subsequent Mormon emigration parties, horses and other animals were raised on the island, accessible at first via a sandbar to the south. The animals were herded north to the California and Oregon Trails in southern Idaho. There the Mormons would trade two fresh animals for four trail-weary ones. The worn beasts of burden would be coaxed to the

Pronghorn antelope on Antelope Island

Back Story

Flash back about 14,000 years. Now try walking where today you find Salt Lake City's streets, or where most Utahns now reside, to the north and south. You would be either drowning or trying frantically to reach the surface of a gigantic, Ice Age body of freshwater we call Lake Bonneville. Nearly 325 miles long, 135 miles wide, and 1,000 feet deep, the lake filled much of what are now the valleys of western Utah, its shores edging into neighboring Nevada and Idaho. Though still large to us, Bonneville's minuscule and shallow primary vestige is the Great Salt Lake. We can add leftovers such as Utah Lake and land-speedsters' favorite Bonneville Salt Flats, if you'd like. The ancient lake is named for Captain Benjamin Bonneville, an early explorer of the West who never actually saw the Great Salt Lake.

According to the Utah Geological Survey, there is evidence that Lake Bonneville's basin has collected water for more than 15 million years. However, beginning about 28,000 years ago, during the cooler, wetter climate of the last ice age, it became a truly great lake, one of the largest in North America. Lake Bonneville stabilized at its greatest extent behind a natural divide near today's Zenda, Idaho, flowing into the Snake River drainage and on to the Pacific Ocean.

Then, about 14,500 years ago, the unconsolidated mud, sand, and boulders of the natural dam in Idaho gave way, causing what geologists call the Bonneville Flood. The incredible cascade scoured the Snake River. At its peak, the flood was equivalent to the average flow of all of our modern rivers combined. Lake Bonneville's level

island for rehab, and the traders realized a profit. Later, homesteaders and miners tested their fortitude and luck on the island, but ultimately it was all purchased by the Island Improvement Co., later the Island Ranching Co., which raised cattle and sheep here for a century.

● The path through the little museum winds around exhibits and to the east. Exit into the high, spacious sheep-shearing barn for a look around. Bison dominate Antelope Island today. Cattle were the ranch's mainstay when the state of Utah bought the entire island from the Anschutz Land and Livestock Co. in 1981. But at one time Garr dropped 375 feet, then found equilibrium again, before climate change ended the Ice Age. The region warmed, precipitation dwindled, and by 11,500 years ago drying Lake Bonneville was comparable to the modern Great Salt Lake. Terrace lines on the Wasatch Mountains, on foothills, and on Antelope and other islands represent periods when the ancient lake stabilized. These are the Bonneville, Stansbury, Gilbert, and other shorelines.

Great Salt Lake's surface level has repeatedly risen and fallen since mountain men,

explorers, and pioneers first saw it in the 19th century. Native people, of course, traveled its shores and used its resources for hundreds of years before that era. The lake was at its lowest in 1963, by which time it had lost about 44 percent of its modern surface area. It rose dramatically during the soggy early 1980s, threatening highways, rail lines, and industry, but again withdrew in the early 2000s. The cycle continues, while we walk city streets, among houses and skyscrapers, and along rural paths, all of which would have once been buried in the depths of Lake Bonneville.

Ranch and Antelope Island were parts of the largest sheep operation in the West. In the mid-1930s, 10,000 of the animals grazed here in the spring and were sheared on a northside platform in one of the world's earliest mechanized operations. Once fleeced, sheep would slip via trap doors into pens below.

● Exit to the south, and turn left toward the corrals, past a silo, where grain was stored before being fed to the livestock or sold. Horses are still kept here on occasion. Stroll west to the open-faced shelters. Here you'll find machinery of the past. Walls and additions bear witness to the corrals' evolution, from stone walls, wooden posts, and milled timber to the corrugated iron of the 20th century. In farrowing pens, sows would be caged and piglets could suckle without being crushed by their gigantic moms. At one spot you may come across lumpy clumps of adobe clay that resemble bricks. Schoolchildren on field trips are often brought here to see what it's like to make adobe, and the results of their amateur labors are what you see.

- Return southeast to the silo you passed near the barn and continue east along the corral fence line, lined with old trucks and antique farm machinery, all well worth a look and perhaps a photo or two. This open field is used for public events, including the annual Memorial Day weekend Cowboy Legends Poetry and Music Gathering.

- Turn left, as the corral fence ends, to walk north into an area called the boneyard. This is the ranch trash dump. Beside the fence is a concrete "dip tank." Ranch hands filled the trough with a mix of creosote and pesticides. Sheep were funneled through the dip to kill ticks and other parasites, and to seal shearing nicks and cuts. Nearby and scattered about are piles of refuse, including broken or obsolete equipment. Several artifacts have been rescued for display around the grounds and in the small museum.

- Return to the barn and orientation area, to the southwest. Outside the barn's southeast corner is an antique sheep camp—a wagon trailer-home. The wagon followed the sheep as they were herded from ranch to grazing areas in the mountains both east and south of the Great Salt Lake. This was the sheepherder's home, with a bed, a stove, shelving, and cupboards. Step inside to see how you'd like this life.

- Stroll south to the ranch house—the oldest pioneer structure in Utah still on its original foundation. As viewed from the front porch, Garr's original adobe-walled house is on the left (south). An obvious line marks the spot where an addition was made with different adobe bricks in the 1870s, in the middle. The northernmost cinder-block section is a shower room for the ranch workers. This was the foreman's house from 1848 to 1981. The exterior and interior reflect its expansion over almost a century and a half.

- Step though a door south of the shower room, just north of center, and you've time-traveled to 1973, when the Anschutz company owned the island. The floors are linoleum. The kitchen had gas, electricity, and appliances of the era—and a few older examples are in the utility room behind it, including a gasoline-powered washing machine.

- Through an entryway to the left (south) is the dining room. Here, during the mid-20th century, family and ranch hands would eat all their meals and, in the evening, play games. The furnishings reflect the era of the 1940s, with an old-style radio and phonograph. A lean-to section at the back of the ranch house offered space for bedrooms, one of which is called Max's Room, for Max Harward. Harward grew up on the ranch, the son of foreman J. B. Harward, and wrote a short memoir of those days, titled "Where the Buffalo Roam."

- The last large room, again to the left (south), is the living room. It is the oldest part of the house. Its décor is a mix of eras, but it is meant to convey the time of Fielding Garr himself: a replica of a Mormon couch, which could be pulled out to make a bed; a wood-burning fireplace; and so on. Guides often suggest visitors search for silver that seems out of place. Look closely at the devices from which the curtain rods hang. They are silverware, bent spoons and forks, nailed into place. This room was later used as a master bedroom, and to the back are two more bedrooms, one with a brass bed, dating it to after the Transcontinental Railroad arrived in Utah in 1869, for it likely would have been too heavy for a wagon-train journey. The other room's bed has no mattress, but rather a rope web for support. Quilted coverings and old-fashioned images on the walls add yet more flavor from the past.

- Step outside the ranch house, east to the porch via the living room's outdoor entrance. Walk east through the quaint yard. To your left is the bunkhouse. Originally an adobe brick structure, it was later covered with concrete and is now painted white. The upper level has beds for ranch hands; cold storage was possible in the cellar. An open spot just beyond, to the east, once was the site of the ranch's long-gone icehouse. Another few steps east, and you've come to the springhouse, dating to the 1880s. Spring water still bubbles up here into a dark pool. The cold water and air circulation allowed those living on the ranch to store milk, cheese,

Fielding Garr ranch house

and other perishables here, where they floated on a little raft. Even when summer temperatures outside rise above 90 or even 100 degrees Fahrenheit, the springhouse remains a cool cave.

● The spring feeds a tree-shaded pool outside, to the east. Watercress grows thick in the water, the source of bucketfuls used for cooking and washing in the ranch house. The grove is a tangle of trunks and branches, though today bison sometimes make their way into the thicket. And occasionally the area is roped off from visitors, so nesting owls can raise their young in some semblance of peace and privacy.

● The formal walk ends here. Return to the parking lot, to the west, behind the ranch house. Or, the Fielding Garr Ranch precincts are larger and open to wandering. Fields to the south are used for camping, but only during a Memorial Day weekend festival and during the annual autumn roundup of Antelope Island's bison herd. This is when, like ranch animals of yesteryear, they are herded into corrals (on the island's north side, nowadays) for inoculations and culling. The roundup is quite a sight: horsemen and horsewomen flushing the bison from fields and hideaways, four-wheel-drive vehicles adding more convincing force to the migration and helicopters buzzing overhead in search of bison trying to evade the parade. Past and present merge at Fielding Garr Ranch on Great Salt Lake's Antelope Island.

POINTS OF INTEREST (START TO FINISH)

Antelope Island State Park and **Fielding Garr Ranch** stateparks.utah.gov/parks/antelope-island, 4528 W. 1700 South, 801-773-294

Island Buffalo Grill Bridger Bay beach, Antelope Island, 801-528-8080

ROUTE SUMMARY

1. Start at the Fielding Garr Ranch parking lot, walking downhill and east, around the blacksmith shop, and slightly north to the barn, which houses the orientation museum.
2. Exit the museum's northern door into the sheep barn.
3. Leave the barn via the eastern portal, turning left to head north past a grain silo.
4. Turn left to stroll west along the corral fences to the corral's long shed.

5. Return east to the silo and continue slightly west, then east, past antique vehicles along the corral's south side.

6. Turn left and north to the ranch's boneyard, or dump.

7. Return west to the barn and the sheep camp wagon on its southeast corner.

8. Cross an open area south to the ranch house and enter its kitchen through a door just north of the structure's midsection.

9. Exit the ranch house via its living room outside door, to walk south past the bunkhouse and the spring house to a grove of trees around the spring's pool.

10. End the walk by returning to the parking lot, or continue strolling the fields at your leisure.

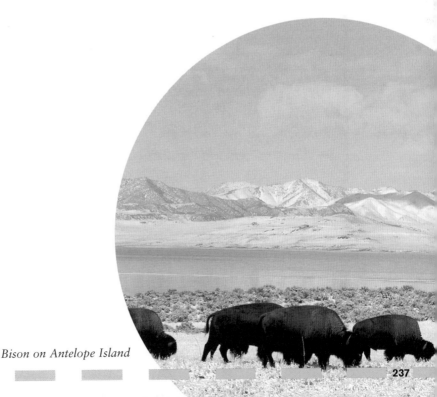

Bison on Antelope Island

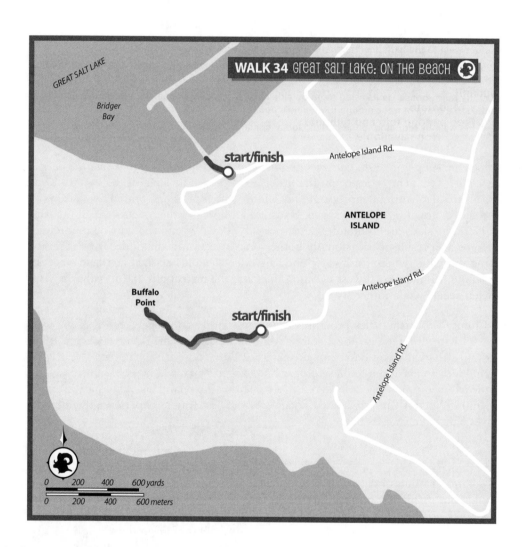

GREAT SALT LAKE

Bridger
Bay

WALK 34 Great Salt Lake: on the Beach

start/finish

Antelope Island Rd.

**ANTELOPE
ISLAND**

Antelope Island Rd.

**Buffalo
Point**

start/finish

Antelope Island Rd.

Antelope Island Rd.

0   200   400   600 yards
0   200   400   600 meters

34 Great Salt Lake: On the Beach

BOUNDARIES: **Bridger Bay, Buffalo Point**
DISTANCE: **0.4 mile on Great Salt Lake's Bridger Bay beach; 0.8 mile round-trip to Buffalo Point summit**
DIFFICULTY: **Moderate**
PARKING: **Free parking lots and pullouts**
PUBLIC TRANSIT: **None available**

How does the song go? "*Oh, give me a home where the buffalo roam/Where the deer and the antelope play. . . .*" The lyrics begin the official, child-friendly song of the state of Kansas, but the words are also entirely appropriate for Utah's Antelope Island State Park. Bison, pronghorn antelope, coyotes, bighorn sheep, birds, and a host of other creatures call the island home. Here the skies are, quite often, "not cloudy all day," and the only discouraging words might come as a result of occasionally bothersome insects and stinky decaying vegetation along the shoreline, where freshwater and saltwater wetlands clash. The island's access point is only about 40 miles northwest of Salt Lake City, the metropolis and its suburbs visible from what seems like another world.

Davis County's tourism office promotes Antelope Island as "a rugged blend of the western outdoors," with dramatic geology, rolling hills, and free-roaming American bison. The setting is essentially a Great Basin desert: open space surrounded by the forbidding Great Salt Lake. Minus modern roads and a few buildings, Antelope has changed little from its early days, when the Mormon pioneers considered this to be fine rangeland, as well as a recreational haven, and dubbed it Church Island. Today it is the best way to experience the inland lake that gives Salt Lake City its name.

Antelope Island, accessible via a 7.2-mile paved causeway from Syracuse, north of Salt Lake City, encompasses 28,022 acres, making it by far the largest isle in the Great Salt Lake. It is approximately 15 miles long and 4.5 miles wide. Most of Antelope is in the 4,300-foot elevation range, but its highest point, Frary Peak, tops out at 6,596 feet above sea level. The island offers a quick escape from the urban hubbub, with sightseeing drives, walking, hiking, biking, camping, horseback riding, and, yes, a visit to a sandy beach. From the incredible sunsets visible atop Buffalo Point to wading or floating in the Great Salt Lake, Antelope is worth a visit for a variety of walks. Sandy beaches, shower facilities, and picnic pavilions are available at Bridger Bay.

Yes, there are insects. Among them are annoying but harmless midges and gnats, and brine flies that do not bite but fly in hazy flocks near the lake's edges, where brine shrimp (the saline lake's major life-form) also litter the shore. Seasonally (late spring and into fall), there are tiny biting flies, often called no-see-ums for their stealth, and there can be biting mosquitoes. Bug repellent is suggested. Antelope Island has a visitor center and museum, snugly built on a hillside above the causeway; a marina; and a single little eatery, Island Buffalo Grill, open seasonally with varying hours, on Bridger Bay.

Because this most rewarding access to the Great Salt Lake shore is a distance from Salt Lake City proper, we suggest pairing two options for simple walks: white-sand Bridger Bay and rocky prominence Buffalo Point. Another route is described in Walk 33, which covers Fielding Garr Ranch, to the southeast. An island visit will introduce you to several other walking and hiking possibilities.

- From Salt Lake City, drive north on I-15 about 24 miles, and take Exit 332 (Layton-Syracuse). Head west about 6 miles on Antelope Dr. (UT 108 and 127). There is a $9 entrance fee for Antelope Island State Park. After the gate, travel 7.2 miles across the causeway, which slices across the Great Salt Lake. Try not to be discouraged by the "lake stink" you might encounter during the causeway's first mile. The odor is caused by decaying material along the mudflats and vanishes once open lake water is reached. The smell is rarely obvious on Antelope Island. Upon reaching the island's northeastern tip, fork right. After proceeding just over 1 mile on the winding road, consider taking the short side road to the visitor center (open 9 a.m.–6 p.m. in summer). Otherwise, travel another 0.6 mile on the paved road (a total of 1.7 miles from the island's tip) to the day-use area of Bridger Bay. Note that if you spot any of the free-roaming buffalo on the island, give them room; do not approach the wild animals.

- Park in a lot at Bridger Bay, near one of the many pavilions. Walk west down to the Great Salt Lake shoreline. After all, how can you truly claim to have walked Salt Lake City without at least touching the briny lake that gave the city its name? Lake levels have recently been on the rise, following nearly a decade of drought. The walk to the water from the parking area has been about 350 yards—downhill, through loose sand, for about 100 yards, followed by another 50 yards on sand and rocks. The remaining

150 yards to the water traverse mudflats and sometimes bug-infested vegetation. Look for a well-worn path through this patch. Tennis shoes, sandals, or flip-flops are preferable to traveling barefoot here.

- You can wade or swim after reaching the water. However, you can't sink. Diving is not recommended, nor is submerging—the salty water will sting your eyes. Before World War II, "floating like a cork" each summer at the Great Salt Lake was as common as going to movies is today. "Try to sink" and "Come on in; the water's fine—you can't sink" were among the catchphrases of the Victorian era. Mormon Church leader and pioneer Wilford Woodruff believed the Great Salt Lake should have been named the eighth wonder of the world. Indeed, Utahns did more than name their city (originally Great Salt Lake City) after this large body of water—they seemed to have an instant love for it. As early as July 27, 1847—days after arriving in the Salt Lake Valley—some tried floating in it. Pioneers described the sensation as something akin to bobbing like a pickle or an empty bottle. Eight bathing resorts sprang up around the eastern and southern shores between 1870 and 1893, all now faded into history.

- If you do venture into the water, you will likely get sand and salt on your body. The salt content of the Great Salt Lake can be up to 28 percent, versus 3 percent in the earth's oceans. Use the handy shower facilities. An outdoor shower is free; an indoor shower costs $1 (payable only in a quarters slot).

- After a lake-water encounter, drive 0.8 mile south to the next junction and turn left to travel east. Drive another 0.4 mile, where you reach a stop sign. Turn right. Stay right at the next junction and drive southwest a total of 1.2 miles from the stop sign and uphill to the parking lot below

Antelope Island's White Rock Bay

Buffalo Point. The view from the lot, overlooking White Rock Bay to the south, is excellent. Several free viewing scopes are available, if you don't want to hike to the top of Buffalo Point. However, the summit gives you a 360-degree, unobstructed view.

- The moderate Buffalo Point hike is short but steep. It begins at 4,550 feet above sea level and climbs to 4,785, for a gain of 235 feet. It is 0.4 mile one-way. (For contrast, the level of the Great Salt Lake averages 4,200 feet above sea level.) The hike begins on a gravel-dirt trail at the west side of the parking lot. Walk up a steep segment over the first rise, after which the trail levels off for a few hundred yards. Then, after several switchbacks, you reach the summit.

- The Buffalo Point hiking trail has been around since 1969, offering a bird's-eye view of the island's north side. Fast hikers can reach the top in eight minutes. An average time would be 12–15 minutes. The west end of the summit offers excellent views and photo opportunities for the causeway, western Davis County, White Rock Bay, Elephant Head, Bridger Bay, and other isles in the lake, such as Fremont and Egg Islands. Bison are often visible in the area.

- The trail continues west into a rocky area, providing additional exploration and adventure for hearty walkers. Children usually find fun among the hollowed-out rocks and small caves on the south slope, west of the summit. It is also possible to continue west after the main trail fades out, to overlook the island's western shore, or even climb down and walk around the rarely visited beach below.

- After summiting Buffalo Point, simply turn around and return down the same trail to the parking lot, to this walk's beginning.

POINTS OF INTEREST (START TO FINISH)

Antelope Island State Park and **Fielding Garr Ranch** stateparks.utah.gov/parks/antelope-island, 4528 W. 1700 South, 801-773-2941

Island Buffalo Grill Bridger Bay beach, Antelope Island, 801-528-8080

rouTe summary

1. Drive north about 24 miles on I-15 from Salt Lake City, to Exit 332 (Layton-Syracuse).

2. Head west about 6 miles on UT 108/127 (Antelope Dr.).

3. After the entrance gate (fee required), travel 7.2 miles west across the causeway.

4. Upon reaching the northeast tip of Antelope Island, fork right and drive 1.7 miles to the Bridger Bay day-use area.

5. Park at Bridger Bay. Walk west down to the shoreline of the Great Salt Lake.

6. After a walk through sand, rock, and seasonal weeds, reach the lake.

7. Return to the parking lot.

8. Drive 0.8 mile south to the next road junction and turn left to travel east.

9. Drive another 0.4 mile to a stop sign. Turn right. Stay right at the next junction.

10. Drive southwest a total of 1.2 miles from the stop sign, proceeding uphill to the parking lot below Buffalo Point.

11. Walk west up the trail to Buffalo Point's summit. The dirt-gravel path goes 0.4 mile, with several switchbacks, and climbs about 235 vertical feet.

12. Return to the parking lot on the same trail.

13. Drive 2.6 miles on the island's east road, which rejoins the causeway.

connecTing The walks

Connect with Walk 33, on the southeast side of Antelope Island, via the east shore drive.

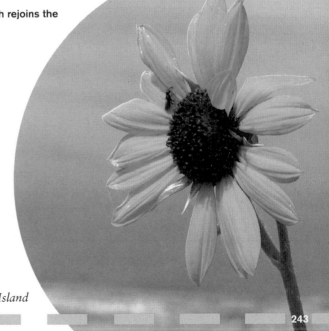

A sunflower on Antelope Island

Appendix 1: WALKS BY THEME

People-Watching

Temple Square (Walk 1)

Main Street (Walk 2)

City Center (Walk 3)

Library Square (Walk 4)

West Downtown (Walk 5)

Liberty Park (Walk 11)

Sugar House Park (Walk 23)

Murray Park (Walk 25)

Arts and Culture

Temple Square (Walk 1)

Main Street (Walk 2)

City Center (Walk 3)

Library Square (Walk 4)

West Downtown (Walk 5)

Capitol Hill (Walk 6)

Memory Grove/City Creek Canyon (Walk 7)

Central City (Walk 10)

Liberty Park (Walk 11)

9th & 9th (Walk 12)

University of Utah (Walk 16)

Fort Douglas (Walk 17)

This Is the Place (Walk 20)

Sugar House (Walk 22)

The Peace Gardens (Walk 29)

Great Salt Lake (Walk 33)

Dining, Shopping, and Entertainment

Temple Square (Walk 1)

Main Street (Walk 2)

City Center (Walk 3)

West Downtown (Walk 5)

Central City (Walk 10)

Liberty Park (Walk 11)

9th & 9th (Walk 12)

Yalecrest Plus (Walk 19)

This Is the Place (Walk 20)

Sugar House (Walk 22)

Murray Park (Walk 25)

Sandy's South Towne (Walk 26)

Lagoon Trail (Walk 32)

Great Salt Lake (Walks 33 and 34)

architectural tours

Temple Square (Walk 1)

Main Street (Walk 2)

City Center (Walk 3)

Library Square (Walk 4)

West Downtown (Walk 5)

Capitol Hill (Walk 6)

East South Temple (Walk 9)

Central City (Walk 10)

Lower Avenues (Walk 13)

Upper Avenues (Walk 14)

University of Utah (Walk 16)

Fort Douglas (Walk 17)

Yalecrest Plus (Walk 19)

This Is the Place (Walk 20)

Sugar House (Walk 22)

Great Salt Lake (Fielding Garr Ranch; Walk 34)

peaceful escapes

Memory Grove/City Creek Canyon (Walk 7)

Ensign Peak (Walk 8)

Liberty Park (Walk 11)

City Cemetery (Walk 15)

Mount Olivet Cemetery (Walk 18)

Sugar House Park (Walk 23)

Parley's Park (Walk 24)

Murray Park (Walk 25)

Temple Quarry (Walk 27)

The Peace Gardens (Walk 29)

serious workouts

Memory Grove/City Creek Canyon (Walk 7)

Ensign Peak (Walk 8)

Bonneville Shoreline (Walk 21)

Jordan River Parkway (Walk 30)

Arrowhead to Germania (Walk 31)

Appendix 2: POINTS OF INTEREST

Beauty and Health

Centered City Yoga 918 E. 900 South, 801-521-9642, centeredcityyoga.com (Walk 12)

The Cosmic Spiral 920 E. 900 South, 801-509-1043, thecosmicspiral.com (Walk 12)

Fairmont Aquatic Center 1044 E. Sugarmont Dr. (2225 South), 801-486-5867, recreation.slco.org/fairmont (Walk 22)

Intermountain Medical Center (flagship hospital) 5121 Cottonwood St., Murray, 801-507-7000, intermountainhealthcare.org/hospitals/imed (Walk 25)

Kura Door Holistic Japanese Spa 1136 E. Third Ave., 801-364-2400, thekuradoor.com (Walk 13)

LDS Hospital Eighth Ave. and C St., 801-408-1100, intermountainhealthcare.org/hospitals/lds (Walk 14)

Cemeteries

Mt. Calvary Cemetery 275 U St., 801-355-2476, mtcalvarycemetery.org (Walk 13)

Mount Olivet Cemetery 1342 E. 500 South, 801-582-2552, mountolivetfriends.org (Walk 18)

Salt Lake City Cemetery 200 N St., 801-596-5020, slcgov.com/publicservices/parks/cemetery.htm (Walk 13)

Educational and Cultural Centers

Clark Planetarium 110 S. 400 West, 801-456-7827, clarkplanetarium.org (Walk 5)

Gallivan Center 239 S. Main, 801-535-6110, slcgov.com/PublicServices/Gallivan (Walk 3)

Highland High School 2166 S. 1700 East, 801-484-4343, highland.slcschools.org (Walk 23)

Hogle Zoo 2600 Sunnyside Ave. (840 South), 801-582-1631, hoglezoo.org (Walk 20)

Jordan High School 95 E. Beetdigger Blvd., Sandy, 801-826-6200, jhs.canyonsdistrict.org/
Jordan_High (Walk 26)

LDS Business College Triad Center, 300 W. North Temple St., 801-524-8100, ldsbc.edu
(Walk 5)

Pioneer Village Lagoon Theme Park Farmington, lagoonpark.com (Walk 32)

Red Butte Garden and Arboretum University of Utah 300 Wakara Way, 801-581-4747,
redbuttegarden.org (Walk 21, near Walk 17)

Salt Lake City Library (Main Library) 210 E. 300 South, 801-524-8200, slcpl.lib.ut.us (Walk 4)

Sprague Public Library 2131 S. 1100 East, 801-594-8640, slcpl.lib.ut.us (Walk 22)

This Is the Place Heritage Park 2601 E. Sunnyside Ave., 801-582-1847, thisistheplace.org
(Walk 20)

Tracy Aviary Liberty Park, 589 E. 1300 South, 801-596-8500, tracyaviary.org (Walk 11)

University of Utah 201 Presidents Circle (100 South and 1500 East), 801-581-7200,
utah.edu (Walk 16)

ENTERTAINMENT AND NIGHTLIFE

Abravanel Hall (home of the Utah Symphony and Utah Opera) 123 W. South Temple St.,
801-533-5626, utahsymphony.org (Walk 3)

Ballet West (Capitol Theatre) 50 W. 200 South, 801-869-6900, balletwest.org (Walk 5)

Broadway Center Cinemas (Salt Lake Film Society) 111 E. Broadway (300 South),
saltlakefilmsociety.org (Walk 4)

Calvin L. Rampton Salt Palace Convention Center 100 S. West Temple St., 801-534-4777,
visitsaltlake.com/saltpalace (Walk 3)

Capitol Theatre (Utah Opera, Ballet West, Broadway in Utah productions) 50 W. 200 S.,
877-686-5366, capitol.theatresaltlakecity.com (Walk 3)

The Depot Club (Union Pacific Depot at The Gateway), 13 N. 400 West, 801-456-2800,
depotslc.com (Walk 5)

EnergySolutions Arena (events, concerts, and home of the NBA's Utah Jazz)
301 W. South Temple St., 801-325-2000, energysolutionsarena.com (Walk 5)

Gallivan Center (concerts, festivals, events, park) 239 S. Main St., 801-535-6110, slcgov.com/publicservices/gallivan (Walks 2 and 4)

Kingsbury Hall 1395 E. Presidents Circle, 801-581-7100, kingsburyhall.org (Walk 16)

KUTV station 299 S. Main St., Suite 150, 801-839-1234, connect2utah.com (Walk 3)

Lagoon Theme Park 375 Lagoon Drive, Farmington, 801-451-8000, lagoonpark.com (Walk 32)

Megaplex 12 at The Gateway (movies) 165 S. Rio Grande St., 801-304-4636, megaplextheatres.com (Walk 5)

Megaplex 17 at Jordan Commons (movies) 9400 S. State St., Sandy, 801-304-4577, megaplextheatres.com (Walk 26)

The Park Center 202 E. Murray Park Ave., Murray, 801-284-4200, murray.utah.gov (Walk 25)

Pioneer Memorial Theater (live professional theater) University of Utah, 300 S. 1400 East, 801-581-6961 (Walk 16)

Post Theatre 245 S. Fort Douglas Blvd., 801-587-1000 (Walk 17)

Rio Tinto Stadium (Real Salt Lake Major League Soccer League, concerts) 9256 S. State St., Sandy, 801-727-2700, riotintostadium.com (Walk 26)

Rose Wagner Performing Arts Center (dance, plays, events) 138 W. 300 South, slccfa.org/venues/rose-wagner-performing-arts-center (Walk 5)

Salt Lake County Ice Center 5201 S. Murray Park Lane, Murray, 801-270-7280, countyice.slco.org (Walk 25)

Seven Peaks Waterpark (formerly Raging Waters) 1200 W. 1700 South, 801-972-3300, ragingwatersutah.com (Walk 30)

South Towne Exposition Center 9575 S. State St., Sandy, 801-565-4490, southtowneexpo.com (Walk 26)

Studio 600 Dance Club 26 E. 600 South, 801-355-9860, mystudio600.com (Walk 4)

Tavernacle Social Club 201 E. 300 South, 801-833-0570, tavernaclenightclub.com (Walk 4)

The Tower Theatre (Salt Lake Film Society) 876 E. 900 South, 801-321-0310, saltlakefilmsociety.org (Walk 12)

Washington Square (Salt Lake City and County Building; events, festivals, park) 451 S. State St. (Walk 4)

FOOD aND DrINK

A. Ray Olpin Union Building University of Utah, 801-581-7251, union.utah.edu (Walk 16)

Bambara Restaurant 202 S. Main St., 801-363-5454, bambara-slc.com (Walk 2)

Barbacoa Mexican Grill 859 E. 900 South, 801-524-0853, eatbarbacoa.com (Walk 12)

Bar X 155 E. 200 South, 801-532-9114 (Walk 4)

Beehive Pub 128 S. Main, 801-364-4268 (Walk 2)

Blue Lemon 55 W. South Temple, 801-328-2583, bluelemon.com (Walk 3)

Caffé Molise 55 W. 100 South, 801-364-8833, caffemolise.com (Walk 3)

Cafe Shambala 328 E Fourth Avenue, 801-364-8558 (Walk 13)

Caputo's Market and Deli 1516 S. 1500 East, 801-486-6615, caputosdeli.com (Walk 19)

Cedars of Lebanon Restaurant 152 E. 200 South, 801-364-4096, cedarsoflebanonrestaurant.com (Walk 4)

Chuck-A-Rama 744 E. 400 South, 801-531-1123, chuck-a-rama.com (Walk 10)

City Creek Center, East Block (food court) 50 S. State St., shopcitycreekcenter.com (Walk 3)

Cucina Gourmet Deli 1026 E. Second Ave., 801-322-3055, cucinadeli.com (Walk 13)

Cucina Nassi banquets 2155 S. Highland Dr., 801-819-7555, cucinanassi.com (Walk 22)

Cucina Toscana 307 W. Pierpont, 801-328-3463 (Walk 5)

Cummings Studio Chocolates 679 E. 900 South, 801-328-4858 (Walk 12)

Desert Edge Brewery at the Pub Trolley Square, 801-521-8917, desertedgebrewery.com (Walk 10)

Dolcetti Gelato 902 E. 900 South, 801-485-3254, dolcettigelato.com (Walk 12)

Elizabeth's Bakery & Tea Shop 439 E. 900 South, 801-433-1170 (Walk 10)

Este New York Style Pizzaria 156 E. 200 South, 801-363-2366, estepizzaco.com (Walk 4)

Francisco's Mexican Grill 7 E. State St., Farmington, 801-451-0383 (Walk 32)

Fresco Italian Café 1513 S. 1500 East, 801-486-1300, frescoitaliancafe.com (Walk 19)

Great Harvest Bread Co. 905 E. 900 South, 801-328-2323, greatharvest.com (Walk 12)

Hagermann's Bakehouse Café 15 W. South Temple, 801-320-9562, hagermanns.com (Walk 3)

Harmon's Grocery 135 E. 100 South, harmonsgrocery.com (Walk 3)

Hire's Big-H Drive-in 425 S. 700 East, 801-364-4582, hiresbigh.com (Walk 10)

Island Buffalo Grill Bridger Bay beach, Antelope Island, 801-528-8080 (Walks 33 and 34)

Joe's Crab Shack 9400 S. State St., 801-255-9571, joescrabshack.com (Walk 31)

Johnny's on Second (tavern) 165 E. 200 South, 801-746-3334, johnnysonsecond.com (Walk 4)

Jordan Commons Food Court 9400 S. State St., Sandy, jordancommons.com (Walk 26)

Lamb's Grill Cafe 169 S. Main St., 801-364-7166, lambsgrill.com (Walks 2 and 3)

Last Samurai 85 E. 9400 South, 801-568-2888, LastSam.com (Walk 31)

Lion House Pantry Restaurant 63 E. South Temple St., 801-539-3257, templesquarehospitality.com/lionhouse (Walk 1)

Litza's Pizza 716 E. 400 South, 801-359-5352, litzaspizza.com (Walk 10)

London Market 439 E. 900 South, 801-531-7074 (Walk 10)

Mrs. Backer's Pastry Shop 434 E. South Temple St., 801-532-2022, mrsbackers.com (Walk 9)

Market Street Grill 48 W. Market St., 801-322-4668, gastronomyinc.com (Walk 2)

Mazza Café 912 E. 900 South, 801-521-4572, mazzacafe.com (Walk 12)

Mazza Middle Eastern Cuisine 1515 S. 1500 East, 801-484-9259, mazzacafe.com (Walk 19)

Michelangelo's on Main 1325 S. Main St., 801-532-0500 (Walk 2)

The Melting Pot 340 S. Main St., 801-521-6358 (Walk 2)

Naked Fish Bistro 67 W. 100 South, 801-595-8888, nakedfishbistro.com (Walk 3)

The New Yorker 60 W. Market St., 801-363-0166, gastronomyinc.com (Walk 2)

9th South Delicatessen 931 E. 900 South, 801-517-3663 (Walk 12)

The Old Spaghetti Factory 189 Trolley Square, 801-521-0424, osf.com (Walk 10)

Pago Restaurant 878 S. 900 East, 801-532-0777, pagoslc.com (Walk 12)

Pagoda Restaurant 26 E St., 801-355-8155 (Walk 9)

The Paris Bistro 1500 S. 1500 East, 801-486-5585, theparis.net (Walk 19)

Rio Grand Café 270 S. Rio Grand St., 801-364-3302 (Walk 5)

Rodizio Grill 600 S. 700 East, 801-220-0500, rodiziogrill.com/salt-lake-city (Walk 10)

Ruby River Steakhouse 435 S. 700 East, 801-359-3355, rubyriver.com (Walk 10)
85 E. 9400 South, 801-569-1889, rubyriver.com (Walk 31)

Sawadee Thai Cuisine 754 E. South Temple St., 801-328-8424, sawadee1.com (Walk 9)

Skool Lunch Deli & Bakery 136 E. South Temple St., 801-532-5269,
southtemple@skoollunch.com (Walk 9)

Smith's Food and Drug 876 E. 800 South, 801-355-2801, smithsfoodanddrug.com (Walk 12)
402 Sixth Ave., 801-328-1683 (Walk 14)

Thai Garden & Noodle House 868 E. 900 South, 801-355-8899 (Walk 12)

This Is the Place/Jack Mormon Coffee Co. 82 N. E St., 801-359-2979 (Walk 13)

Tony Caputo's Market & Deli 308 W. 300 South, 801-531-8669 (Walk 5)

Tropical Dreams Hawaiian Creamery 928 E. 900 South, 801-359-0986,
tropicaldreamsicecream.com (Walk 12)

Tucci's Cucina Italiano Trolley Corners, 515 S. 700 East, 801-533-9111 (Walk 10)

Washington Square Café 451 S. State St., 801-535-6102 (Walk 4)

Whole Foods Market 544 S. 700 East, 801-924-9060,
wholefoodsmarket.com/stores/trolleysquare (Walk 10)

Wonder Bread Bakery 734 E. 400 South, 801-531-6057 (Walk 10)

X-Wife's Place 465 S. 700 East, 801-532-1954 (Walk 10)

Historical Landmarks and Monuments

Beehive House 67 E. South Temple St., 801-240-2681 (Walk 1)

Devereaux Mansion 340 W. South Temple St., 800-881-5762,
templesquarehospitality.com/mansion/weddings (Walk 5)

East High School 840 S. 1300 East, 801-583-1661, slc.k12.ut.us/schools/high/east (Walk 19)

Exchange Place Boston and Newhouse Buildings, 350 S. Main St. (Walk 2)

Frank E. Moss Federal Courthouse (former U.S. Post Office) 350 S. Main St. (Walk 2)

Kearns Building 136 S. Main St. (Walk 2)

Memorial House and Memory Grove 485 N. Canyon Rd. (Walk 7)

Pony Express site 143 S. Main St. (Walk 2)

Rio Grande Depot 300 S. Rio Grande, 801-533-3500, history.utah.gov/about_us/depot (Walk 5)

Salt Lake City and County Building 451 S. State St., 801-535-6333, slcgov.com/government (Walk 4)

Salt Lake Masonic Temple 650 E. South Temple St., 801-363-2936, wasatchlodge.org (Walk 9)

Trolley Square 500 S. 700 East, 801-521-9877, trolleysquare.com and trolleysquaremerchants.com (Walk 10)

Union Pacific Depot (at The Gateway) South Temple St. and 400 West (Walk 5)

Utah State Capitol 350 N. State St., 801-538-3074, utahstatecapitol.utah.gov (Walk 6)

Utah Governor's Mansion 603 E. South Temple St., utah.gov/governor/mansion (Walk 9)

Utah Travel Council (old Salt Lake City Hall) 300 N. State St., 801-538-1398, travelutah.gov (Walk 6)

Walker Center 179 S. Main St., comre.com/walker_center (Walk 3)

LODGING

Anniversary Inn 678 E. South Temple St., 800-363-4960, anniversaryinn.com/south-temple (Walk 9)

Carlton Hotel Inn & Suites 140 E. South Temple St., 800-633-3500, carltonhotel-slc.com (Walk 9)

Grand America Hotel 555 S. Main St., 800-304-8696, grandamerica.com (Walk 4)

Haxton Manor Bed and Breakfast 943 E. South Temple St., 877-930-4646, haxtonmanor.com (Walk 9)

Homestead Studio Suites 1220 E. 2100 South, 801-474-0771, homesteadhotels.com (Walk 22)

Homewood Suites by Hilton 423 W. 300 South, 801-363-6700, homewoodsuites1.hilton.com (near Walk 4 and Walk 5)

Hotel Monaco 15 W. 200 South, 801-595-0000, monaco-saltlakecity.com (Walk 2)

Little America Hotel 500 South Main St., 800-281-7899, littleamerica.com (Walk 4)

Lagoon RV Park and Campground 375 N. Lagoon Dr., Farmington, 801-451-8100, lagoonpark.com/parkInfo/camping (Walk 32)

Shilo Inn Suites 206 S. West Temple St., 801-521-9500, shiloinns.com (near Walks 2 and 3)

MUSEUMS AND ART GALLERIES

6th Avenue Gallery and Frame Shop 752 E. 6th Ave., 801-359-4604 (Walk 14)

15th Street Gallery 1519 S. 1500 East, 801-468-1515, 15thstreetgallery.com (Walk 19)

Art Access 230 S. 500 West, #125, 801-328-0703 (Walk 5)

The Art Barn (Finch Lane Gallery, Salt Lake Arts Council) Reservoir Park, 1340 E. South Temple St., 801-596-5000, slcgov.com/arts/pages/vizarts.htm (Walk 9)

Art at the Main Salt Lake City Public Library, ground floor, 210 E. 400 South, 801-363-4088 (Walk 4)

Arts of The World Gallery 802 S. 600 East, 801-532-8035 (Walk 10)

Church History Museum The Church of Jesus Christ of Latter-day Saints 45 N. West Temple St., 801-240-3310, lds.org/churchhistory/museum (Walk 1)

Daughters of Utah Pioneers Museum (see Pioneer Memorial Museum below)

Discover Gateway Children's Museum (at The Gateway) 444 W. 100 South, 801-456-5437, discoverygateway.org (Walk 5)

Fort Douglas Museum 32 Potter St., 801-581-1710, fortdouglas.org (Walk 17)

Gilgal Sculpture Garden 749 E. 500 South, gilgalgarden.org (Walk 10)

The Leonardo (museum) 300 S. 500 East, 801-531-9800, theleonardo.org (Walk 4)

Natural History Museum of Utah Rio Tinto Center, University of Utah, umnh.utah.edu (Walk 21)

Olympic Cauldron Park 451 S. 1400 East, 801-581-8849, stadium.utah.edu (Walk 16)

Pioneer Memorial Museum (Daughters of Utah Pioneers) 300 N. Main St., 801-532-6479 ext. 206, dupinternational.org (Walk 6)

Rio Gallery (Rio Grande Depot/Utah Division of State History) 300 S. Rio Grande, 801-533-3582 (Walk 5)

Rockwood Art Studios 1062 and 1064 E. 2100 South, rockwood.shawnrossiter.com (Walk 22)

Salt Lake Art Center (Salt Palace/Abravanel Hall) 20 S. West Temple St., 801-328-4201 (Walk 3)

Sons of Utah Pioneers Building 3301 East 2920 South (on the rim at the southeast side of Parley's Hollow), 866-724-1847, sonsofutahpioneers.org (near Walk 24)

Utah Artist Hands 61 W. 100 South, 801-355-0206 (Walk 3)

Utah Arts Alliance Gallery 127 S. Main St., 801-651-3937 (Walk 2)

Utah Museum of Fine Arts University of Utah, Marcia and John Price Museum Building, 410 Campus Center Dr., 801-581-7332, umfa.utah.edu (Walk 16)

Parks and Gardens

Antelope Island State Park and Fielding Garr Ranch 4528 W. 1700 South, Syracuse, 801-773-2941, stateparks.utah.gov/parks/antelope-island (Walk 33)

Dimple Dell Park 10400 South 1300 East, Sandy (Walk 28)

Eighth South Artesian Well Park 800 South and 500 East (Walk 10)

International Peace Gardens at Jordan Park 1000 S. 900 West (Walk 29)

Jordan River Parkway utah.com/stateparks/jordan_river (Walks 30 and 31)

Liberty Park 1300 South and 700 East (Walk 11)

Lindsey Gardens M St. and 7th Ave. (Walk 14)

Memory Grove N. Canyon Rd. (Walk 7)

Miller Bird Refuge 1500 E. 1050 South, utahbirds.org/counties/saltlake/MillerBirdPark (Walk 19)

Murray Park 5300 S. State St., Murray, 801-264-2614, murray.utah.gov (Walk 25)

Pioneer Park 300 S. 300 West, downtownslc.org/farmers-market (Walk 5)

Popperton Park 1400 E. Popperton Park Way (360 North) (Walk 14)

Red Butte Gardens University of Utah 300 Wakara Way, 801-585-0556, redbuttegarden.org (Walk 21)

Sugar House Garden Center 1610 E. 2100 South, 801-467-1721, sugarhousepark.org (Walk 23)

Sugar House Park 1300 East and 2100 South, 801-467-1721, sugarhousepark.org (Walk 23)

Taufer Park (Madonna tree) 700 S. 300 East (Walk 10)

Tracy Aviary Liberty Park 589 E. 1300 South, 801-596-8500, tracyaviary.org

SHOPPING

Aunt Addys Country Home 58 N. Main St., Farmington, 801-451-6400 (Walk 32)

Cahoots Cards & Gifts 878 E. 900 South, 801-538-0606 (Walk 12)

City Creek Center between South Temple St. and 100 South and West Temple St. and State St., downtownrising.com (Walk 3)

Cobwebs Antiques and Collectibles 1054 E. 2100 South, 801-485-9295 (Walk 22)

The Free Speech Zone 411 S. 800 East, 801-487-2295, freespeechzone.wordpress.com (Walk 10)

The Gateway 18 N. Rio Grande St., 801-456-2000, shopthegateway.com (Walk 5)

Gift Shop at This Is the Place Heritage Park Visitor Center 2601 E. Sunnyside Ave., 801-582-1847 (Walk 20)

Just a Bed of Roses 15 E. State St., Farmington, 801-628-0890, justabedofroses.blogspot.com (Walk 32)

Ken Sanders Rare Books 268 S. 200 East, 801-521-3819, kensandersbooks.com/shop/rarebooks (Walk 4)

The Kings English Bookshop 1511 S. 1500 East, 801-484-9100, kingsenglish.com (Walk 19)

Macy's City Creek Center, East Block, Main St. and 50 South (Walk 3)

Night Flight Comics 210 E. 400 South, 801-532-1188, night-flight.com (Walk 4)

Nordstrom City Creek Center, West Block, West Temple St. and 50 West (Walk 3)

Pottery Barn 552 S. 602 East, 801-322-4050, potterybarn.com (Walk 10)

South Towne Center (shopping mall) 10450 S. State St., Sandy, 801-572-1516, southtownecenter.com (Walk 26)

Sundance Catalog Outlet 2201 S. Highland Dr., sundancecatalog.com (Walk 22)

Trolley Square 500 S. 700 East, 801-521-9877, trolleysquare.com and trolleysquaremerchants.com (Walk 10)

Weller Book Works 607 Trolley Square, 801-328-2586, wellerbookworks.com (Walk 10)

Ski resorts

Alta Ski Resort 801-359-1078, alta.com (Walk 27)

Snowbird Ski and Summer Resort Top of Little Cottonwood Canyon, 800-232-9542, snowbird.com (Walk 27)

Spiritual institutions

Cathedral of the Madeleine 331 E. South Temple St., 801-328-8941, saltlakecathedral.org (Walk 9)

Church History Library, The Church of Jesus Christ of Latter-day Saints 15 E. North Temple St., 801-240-2745, lds.org/churchhistory/library (Walk 1)

Conference Center, The Church of Jesus Christ of Latter-day Saints Northwest corner of North Temple and Main Sts. (Walk 1)

Congregation Kol Ami 2425 Heritage Way (west of Tanner Park), 801-484-1501, conkolami.org (Walk 24)

First Presbyterian Church of Salt Lake 12 C St. (about 380 E. South Temple St.), 801-363-3889, fpcslc.org (Walk 9)

First United Methodist Church 203 E. 200 South, 801-328-8726, firstmethodistslc.org (Walk 4)

Fort Douglas Post Chapel 120 S. Fort Douglas Blvd., 801-587-1000 (Walk 17)

Gilgal Sculpture Garden 749 E. 500 South, gilgalgarden.org (Walk 10)

Holy Trinity Cathedral 279 S. 300 West, 801-328-9681, gocslc.org (Walk 5)

Joseph Smith Memorial Building 52 N. Main St., 801-539-3130, templesquarehospitality.com/jsmb (Walk 1)

St. Mark's Cathedral 231 E. 100 South, 801-322-3400, stmarkscathedral-ut.org (Walk 4)

Temple Square (Salt Lake LDS Temple, Salt Lake Tabernacle, Assembly Hall) Main and South Temple Sts., 801-240-1706, visittemplesquare.com (Walk 1)

Trinity African American Episcopal Church 39 E. 600 South, 801-531-7374 (Walk 10)

White Memorial Chapel 150 E. 300 North, utahstatecapitol.utah.gov (Walk 6)

INDEX

ABOUT THE AUTHORS

Lynn Arave is a native Utahn and a graduate of Weber State University in communications and human performance. He is a retired newspaper reporter who worked as a journalist for more than 31 years. An avid hiker and walker, he currently lives in Layton, Utah, with his wife, LeAnn. They are the parents of four children—Roger, Steven, Elizabeth, and Taylor.

Ray Boren is a lifelong Utahn and professional writer, editor, and photographer. A graduate of the University of Utah in mass communications, he was for 35 years a reporter, feature writer, editor, and ultimately deputy managing editor of a Salt Lake City daily newspaper. His current focus is on photography, free-lance writing, book projects, and travel.

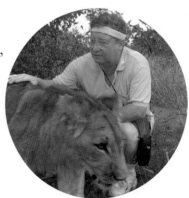

Visit us online at facebook.com/WalkingSaltLakeCity.